Nothing Personal

Disturbing undercurrents in cancer care

MITZI BLENNERHASSETT

Foreword by
Professor KAROL SIKORA

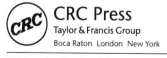

CRC Press
Taylor & Francis Group
Boca Raton   London   New York

CRC Press is an imprint of the
Taylor & Francis Group, an **informa** business

CRC Press
Taylor & Francis Group
6000 Broken Sound Parkway NW, Suite 300
Boca Raton, FL 33487-2742

First issued in hardback 2017

© 2008 Mitzi Blennerhassett
CRC Press is an imprint of Taylor & Francis Group, an Informa business

No claim to original U.S. Government works

ISBN-13: 978-1-84619-010-0 (pbk)
ISBN-13: 978-1-138-45095-0 (hbk)

Visit the Taylor & Francis Web site at
http://www.taylorandfrancis.com

and the CRC Press Web site at
http://www.crcpress.com

Foreword by
Professor Karol Sikora ▬▬

This is a remarkable book. It is the synthesis of the cancer journey of one very unusual person told in both prose and poetry. 'Who'd want to know?' the first poem asks and that sums it all up. Well, we all do of course. Truth is a rationed commodity in modern medicine. Of course we've come a long way from when cancer patients were routinely deceived into thinking they had a cyst or some inflammation. On ward rounds we talked carefully in code – neoplastic change, mitotic activity, anaplasia. These were the euphemisms of the seventies.

Now the word cancer is used freely: on hospital signs, on leaflets and by the media. Indeed it's inescapable in today's complex, consumerist and intrusive world. Pop stars regularly beat cancer and the military metaphors – the war against the disease, collateral damage and the battle at the front line are all pervasive. But the significance of findings of investigations and the true outcomes for an individual with their particular stage, grade and type of cancer are usually shrouded in professional vagueness. This book will surely inspire change.

This year over a quarter million people in Britain will be told they have cancer. Today 1.3 million are living with the disease and this could soar to over 3 million by 2028 because of some remarkable advances on the horizon. There has been an explosion in our molecular understanding and we are now poised to see some incredible advances in prevention, detection and treatment. Cancer will become a chronic illness, joining conditions such as diabetes, heart disease and asthma. These currently impact on how people live but do not inexorably lead to death. Long-term survival will be normal even for patients with cancers that have spread from their primary site. Dramatic progress is likely in all modalities of treatment so leading to increased cure but at a price. Despite all these advances, people living with cancer and also their family and friends all have to learn to live with uncertainty. Here we get a remarkable glimpse of how the author did it.

This is the story of just one person but it is repeated time and time again by many, all over the world. She has a complex but potentially curable cancer from the outset – one that requires a surgical intervention, radiotherapy and chemotherapy to treat optimally. So Mitzi experiences everything. With a young and very active family to look after, she has a lot to live for so how she deals with uncertainty is fascinating. The disruption to her life by the cancer and its treatment is massive and to add to it all she is going through a marital breakdown at the same time. She deals with it all by writing poetry at 3am. I feel it's an incredible privilege to be allowed to follow her journey so closely.

This is essential reading for all who deal with cancer patients – health professionals, politicians, health service developers, carers and, of course, patients themselves. It clearly gives us a distillation of what cancer patients want. We need to create a new network of modern cancer centres where the latest technology in radiotherapy and chemotherapy is seamlessly delivered in a comfortable, welcoming environment. Novel information technology can be used to link the centres so every patient will be monitored to get the best possible treatment.

We have to encourage patients and their families to access information on all aspects of living with cancer. Relaxed information lounges in the centres could provide printed and computer-based access to global knowledge. A future patient-centred, holistic service needs to include complementary medicine which we know improves the quality of many patients' lives during treatment.

We have to value patients' time, so all aspects of care from car parking to drug administration will be carried out as easily and efficiently as possible. Queues and long waiting times need to disappear. Dedicated professionals need to be on hand to explain, guide and assist patients every step of the way. Cancer patients can no longer be service users but valued customers. The way forward is made clear by the usefully referenced discussion sections at the end of each chapter.

For many, cancer is a very lonely experience. We have to recognise the tremendous need for strong support especially during the early phases of treatment. Above all the powerful message of this book is to be honest. Lying, even with the best intentions, simply doesn't work. Trust is an essential component of the vital partnership between patient and professional.

Professor Karol Sikora
February 2008

About the author

Mitzi Blennerhassett has been involved in trying to improve cancer services over almost two decades and is well known in her field. She ran a cancer support group for 12 years, was a member of the Community Health Council for eight years, and began speaking out at a time when the patient voice was not being heard, 'inadvertently' becoming a patient advocate and feisty campaigner. She has been involved in medical education as speaker and 'simulated patient' and has given presentations internationally.

National involvement has included sitting on the Department of Health Pathology Modernisation Oversight Strategy Group and work with the National Audit Office. Her experiences of working alongside patient-centred clinicians (particularly chairing the Lay Advisory Committee of the Royal College of Pathologists, and membership of the Royal College of General Practitioners' Patient Partnership Group) became a turning point in laying her own ghosts to rest. She would like to see patient involvement saturating medical education: for 'Them' and 'Us' to become 'We'.

Mitzi is a member of the Society of Authors' *Medical Writers Group* and has run workshops on therapeutic writing, as well as relaxation and visualisation. She currently contributes to the work of a research group, two Cancer Network User Groups, and many national cancer charities. She also runs painting classes for members of the University of the Third Age.

She enjoys white Stilton, white port and black humour.

*For my children, Finn, Grant, Barley and Dugan,
with thanks for bringing such fun to my life.*

*Also, for my long-suffering friends, for those
whom cancer has touched and with special thanks to
everyone who works to improve cancer services.*

'Truth hurts, but deceit hurts more.'
Lesley Fallowfield

PART I

Author's note ▬▬▬

"How are you?" "Fine!" – "How are you?" "Fine!" Other people might have been psychologically affected by cancer, but not me. My own ghosts were well battened down.

Then came the poems, involuntarily flooding out at 3.00am, night after night. Not a poet's poems, just 'a cancer patient's release', the product of an unquiet mind with no pretence at literary merit, written when I was still very fragile: a search for meaning in nonsense, order in chaos. Indebtedness competed with unmet needs in endless circles, while guilt barred any resolution. I felt guilty for not communicating effectively, for resenting the plastic smiles, the kindly-meant paternalism; for needing more than they could give. I felt an overwhelming sadness that my experiences could be so bad, when everyone seemed to be doing their best. In the end, I could feel nothing. But within these lines lay a call for acknowledgement and change. These were my feelings, laid bare.

I was encouraged to keep writing when someone who read my efforts felt enabled to set down her own experiences and cried for the first time since losing a child to cancer ten years previously.

I wanted to use the poems to promote understanding of the patient's perspective but, although medical journals later published articles about my experiences, this was the early 1990s and feelings were not allowed. So I wrote, and I cried, and I shut them away.

Later involvement in health services prompted me to dust them off and they have been used in medical education, to inform planners of a new cancer centre and to raise money for charity. Therapeutic poems may communicate what could not be spoken but, by their spontaneity, may leave some questions unanswered for the reader. I hope this book will fill the gaps.

Poetry can be very emotive. When linked to experiences associated with a caring profession, it may be distinctly challenging and difficult to accept. I hope the reader will look beyond the emotion to the issues raised. My intention is to 'do no harm'.

Today's patients continue to raise the same issues, but clinicians are now being encouraged to get in touch with their own feelings, so perhaps my story will be useful in helping them acknowledge the emotional and psychological disturbances that can affect both patient and doctor.

Chapter 1

Cancer Country
How was it for me in Cancer Country?
Well, who'd want to know? And whatever for?
It's all been written many times over
What a bore
But while the theme tune sounds familiar
Everyone has a different score

A lone gull makes its way across the sky, battling against the wind. Unremarkable enough, yet it's enough to whisk me back through time. Along with certain words and phrases, this bird has assumed a particular significance in my life with the power to endure through eighteen years; to mock my defences; to open old wounds.

The day that brown envelope dropped through the letter-box was similarly unremarkable, but it was the butterfly that would create a tornado. True, my stomach tightened as I read the hospital letter, but that was to be expected. I was on unfamiliar ground. But there were no warning bells as I noted down the appointment in my diary. No omens. No 'signs of ill portent'. Not a black raven in sight! Yet it heralded the most momentous event in my life. Soon, a spattering of red-ringed reminders would deface the calendar, prophetically resembling red-rimmed eyes. The world would tilt, a chasm would open and for a moment time would stand still. There would be mind-battering aftershocks; life-shattering changes. Memories would become re-categorised 'before' or 'after'. And a year that should have been ordinary would become a milestone, a memory gauge more powerful than birthdays, marriages or deaths.

You'd have thought the gods might at least have given me a hint of what was to come.

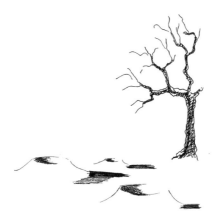

Figure 1.1 Cancer Country.

Chapter 2

In 1961 I'd married a tea-planter and moved to a remote corner of north-east India bordering Nepal and Bhutan. At that time, political unrest, increasing attacks on ex-patriate estate managers and rising taxes had already persuaded several English families to leave the plantations and return 'home'. Two years later the Chinese invaded, advancing to a point just 100 miles away. Women and children were evacuated to Calcutta in huge RAF transport planes. With bi-annual leave due and a four month old baby to consider, we decided to make our return to England permanent.

After becoming International Director for a poultry company, then running his own export business for a while, my husband became an agricultural consultant and worked mainly abroad, mostly for the United Nations' Food and Agricultural Organisation. In India I had reared wild animals; in England I raised 4 children (and often joked that the experiences were not dissimilar). Much of the time I was virtually a 'single mum' and learned to cope with crises ranging from spiders to greenstick fractures. But, in consultancy, 'rest' times meant 'lean' times and the offer of full-time employment persuaded us north in 1982.

Tucked into a corner of the sprawling village green, our new home was a small cottage boasting a range of brick loose boxes and outhouses. But it was the land that 'sold' it to us: six acres of gently sloping fields including a natural pond, bounded on three sides by a 'green lane' and quiet, narrow country roads. We had not only bought a smallholding, we had bought a peninsula!

Downsizing was a squeeze, even though two sons had already left home. Our thirteen year old daughter gallantly put up with a bedroom that would have battered the brains of a swung cat, willing to let her seven year old computer-buff brother lay claim to the larger one, because her interests lay outside: she had a beautiful, new, dapple-grey pony, 'Romany'. The rest of the family consisted of Brachet, a bouncy labrador, Fizzie, an exuberant terrier and Hepzibah the goat, who definitely did not identify with livestock: although her job description included devouring tussocks disdained by the horses, she preferred to demolish hedges. A young tabby cat made her home with us, we had successions of puppies and kittens, reared hens, ducks, geese and calves and kept a companion pony to 'bring on' and sell to offset expenses. This was the 'good life' that so many people sought.

The rural location offered few job opportunities for me that fitted in with chauffeuring children to their schools and activities. I worked as a playgroup supervisor, then a school teaching assistant. When my GP wanted a replacement receptionist for her single GP rural practice just two miles from home, I jumped at the chance.

Our daughter's precocious riding talent deserved to be nurtured and, with progression from ponies to horses, we entered the serious world of affiliated competitions and travelled ever further a-field. It was rare to return home without trophies. My roles as driver, part-time groom, jump-judge and dressage writer became increasingly demanding – and a safety valve in our marriage. Caught up in the excitement of the competition, I was able to switch off for a few hours and live another life.

When my husband was made redundant he returned to consultancy work, but periods of joblessness increased. Even as our marriage deteriorated, I could at least take comfort in my surroundings, the children, the animals . . . and then the sky fell in.

Chapter 3

'Going to the loo, doing a poo, passing a motion, opening one's bowels, defecating' – we all do it, but discussing anything connected with bodily waste is one of society's taboos. Grannie used to clutch me close with her claw-like hand and whisper, "Have you had your bowels open?" My own generation's attitude is hardly less inhibited.

A few years after moving north, I experienced worrying symptoms of pain and bleeding when defecating. A consultant pumped air up my backside for a better view, decided the cause was a small, post childbirth haemorrhoid, proclaimed it 'nothing to worry about' and advised eating more bran. But the barium meal x-ray he arranged, 'just to make sure', was never carried out because I could not give the clinic the precise date of my last period. Although I explained I could not be pregnant, since my husband had been working abroad for the previous three months, they still refused to do it! The unjust implication lit my fuse, already shortened by fear and the stress of the previous twenty-four hours. (The evening before, I'd felt compelled to go ahead with a planned riding event, rather than mention the hospital appointment to my daughter, but I'd had to take loathsome cod liver oil and riding schools are not known for their toilet facilities. I had worried all evening in case I had sudden urgency and an 'accident'.)

Uncharacteristically, and because I was so stressed, I said if they did not do the procedure, I would not be coming back. They still refused! This apparent lack of urgency confirmed the consultant's reassurances.

Weeks later, he wrote to me suggesting it would be a good idea to have the procedure, but the hospital did not send another appointment and I was too fearful to contact them. (My mother had undergone 4 operations for 'stones' in her kidneys and her experiences had left me frightened of hospitals.) They'd said there was 'nothing to worry about' so I believed them. False reassurances worked too well, bran helped the symptoms subside and I just fell off the end of a list. However, the pain had returned and by December 1989 has become so fierce it can no longer be ignored.

It's not until the rush of Christmas has passed that I feel able to focus on my problem and tell my GP boss about the increasing pain and also the lump in my groin, discovered two days earlier. The practice has changed hands, but is still run by a lone, female GP. After taking a look at my backside, she tells me it's anal warts, but she'll refer me to a surgeon 'just in case'.

"I thought it might have been something serious, like cancer," I say, sheepishly, relief flooding through me.

"Huh? Oh no! Nothing like that!" she laughs and tells me to get dressed. I remind her about the lump. After feeling it and asking me to cough, she pronounces it a 'small hernia'. I'm amazed. How long has it been there? Had it been caused by hauling the heavy horse-trailer around in the yard recently? Why hadn't I felt it happen? Driving home, I can't help wondering why she had not done an internal rectal examination.

When I receive a hospital appointment for the next week, I'm not alarmed, assuming they give NHS employees priority. After carrying out a rectal examination, the consultant says he doesn't think it's anything to worry about, but they will take a look under general anaesthetic 'just to make sure'. I guess they are just taking every precaution. When he notices the lump in my groin, I tell him my GP said it's a hernia.

"Yes, I think she's probably right," he confirms and arranges for me to be admitted in two days time.

I wake from the general anaesthetic expecting to be told whether or not I'll need an operation for haemorrhoids, but all I get is smiles. Everything must be fine, or the nurse wouldn't look so cheerful and they'd be discussing operations – wouldn't they? It's going to be a two-day wait until the next appointment. *Why don't they tell me now?* Anyway, I console myself, the lack of urgency confirms the absence of malignancy. I have a lot to learn about hospitals and the way they function.

My experience of unnecessary pain begins next day when I try to have my bowels open. It's so acute I have to tighten my bottom muscles to prevent passing anything. They'd said they would 'just take a look', but I realise they must have taken a biopsy. Nobody had asked my permission, or even informed me afterwards. They must have known the general anaesthetic would slow things down and cause constipation, but nobody thought about giving me anything to counteract it. Nobody thought about my pain. *Nobody thought*. It's a hard lesson, one I am to recall several times in the near future.

Lactulose syrup sorts out my problem. I don't realise the vile stuff is soon to become part of my life. This morning I'm just glad it makes normal function possible.

DISCUSSION

How did you feel when they refused to do the procedure?
Outraged. If they could accept a patient's word about their known period date, why couldn't they take my word about not being pregnant?

How did you feel when you realised they were not going to give you the results of their investigations straight away?
Demoralized. It seemed cruel to cause such stress. I did not know they had to wait for pathology results.

How did you feel when you realised they had taken a biopsy?
Duped, vulnerable and frightened by their disregard for my pain. I knew nothing about giving consent for procedures.

Why do you think the surgeon confirmed the hernia diagnosis?
He probably thought the GP had been 'protecting' me by calling it a hernia, although this was not the case. By going along with this, taking the easy road, he did not have to deal with my emotions.

What needed to change?
Honesty, rather than false reassurance, would allow patients to understand their situation and make informed choices.

Hospital staff need to *listen* to patients[1] and be flexible. Rather than put the onus on me to take action, a new appointment, perhaps backed by a supportive phone call, would have encouraged concordance.

Patients need to know in advance:
» why tests or investigations of any kind need to be carried out
» how long they will have to wait for test results
» what results might mean.

Consent should be obtained before biopsies are taken.

The need for pain relief during and after investigative procedures should be considered routinely and discussed with patients beforehand.

The hospital pharmacy could have provided Lactulose syrup on the ward to take home.

Chapter 4

Being kind to be cruel
Freeze-dried moment
History-changing
Time set waiting, gears set grating
Walls of glass come slamming down, setting me apart

Now there is 'before' and 'after'
Stark. Oppressive.
Brightness. Dark.
'Neural gridlock' in the footlights' glare
Yet all my senses scream, fine-tuned,
At your words, lasering gelatinous air

Thoughts fragmented, deconstructed
Humiliation!
How naïve to have believed
Duped!

Disbelief at the deceit
Incredulity
That you should choose *this* way to break the news

Backtrack
Replay holds no answer
Not even a hint
All saved for today
Confidence shattered, elusive as trust
The trust that I'm craving
Now, an absolute, tangible *'must'*
But you don't seem to know what you've taken away

Without a firm grounding, I'm hanging mid-air
But faultless detachment frees you from care
Control and delivery done with precision
Maximum impact, exquisite incision

While I must be looked upon with derision
– You've known all along and not shared

False reassurances, smiles on a tiger
Worked like a charm
But you don't seem to know you're compounding the harm

As from another world I see
A vulture, squat upon your chair
Uttering unspeakable things
To me

My world upended, devastated
Intrinsic normality, to you
The dog-eared script, the repetition
Understandable boredom, hard to disguise
But it's *my life*
And even now you're not telling it straight

No comfort there
A corridor, with wooden chair
Busy people passing through

"A cup of tea?" A nice hot cup of tea!
I could have laughed
If only I could have cried

I step carefully, avoiding outstretched legs and bags, and squeeze into the crowded waiting area, surrounded by people, but alone. Silence rules, eye contact is avoided. None of us wants to be here. Some flip half-heartedly through out-dated magazines, affecting a sudden interest in everything from cars and puddings, to sex, before consigning them back to the untidy pile. Dog-eared posters compete for space on a notice-board half hidden by patients' heads. There are no helpful leaflets. Thankfully I've brought a calming distraction and try several times to immerse myself in the pages of Mary Wesley's 'Not That Sort of Girl',[2] but with only partial success.

A friend once described her experience of a haemorrhoid operation in colourful detail. ". . . Afterwards, they put a tube up your bottom and turn it every day, twisting it against the raw flesh." I cringe at the memory, hoping there are more humane methods these days. *Keep thinking positive. I'm just here for results. Perhaps I won't need an operation at all.* My name rings out, cutting through the silence and I'm on my feet and on my way.

He's sitting behind a desk, reading my notes. He has yet to acknowledge my presence. I sit down uninvited, still buoyed up by lingering remnants of Mary Wesley's humour, nervously hoping my smile will convey confidence. *Maybe it's something that can be cured with drugs, or diet. Yes or no? Please tell me quickly – the thought of being cut open is terrifying.* He ignores me.

"Good morning," I offer, tentatively, a mouse faking bravery. He looks up, but returns neither my greeting nor my smile – and his words freeze time.

"Yes, well, you *have* a tumour." The dry delivery as nonchalant and bored as a weather forecast.

The words land like a physical blow, delivered with ramrod efficiency. Ratchets slip in the clockwork of my brain. Falteringly, I try to absorb a statement that contradicts everything they have already told me. *Accent on the 'have' – 'just as we'd thought – surely you'd realised?'*

What of the smiling reassurances, the outright denial? I'm caught completely off-guard. The shock is total – the effect, pulverising, devastating. Brutal delivery achieves maximum impact. I feel my smile drop away. *'The smile was wiped from her face . . .' How can I be thinking like this . . . at a time like this!* Mangled thoughts compete. *A tumour . . . Why doesn't he say 'cancer'? I am going to die. How long . . .?*

A wave of overwhelming incredulity and humiliation slams into me. *They've known this all along. They have been limiting information about my body as if I was not competent to deal with it! No previous discussion about possibilities or probabilities. No word of warning. But this is their job: they must be telling people they have cancer every day. Surely they have perfected the best way of doing it? Why have they chosen this cruel way to tell me – stringing me along until the last minute?*

Futile questions. Turmoil. It's incomprehensible. Will not compute! I am going to die! Do I have months – weeks – less? What about my children? I wait, paralysed, expecting words of comfort. But things get worse.

"Did you think you might have a tumour?"

The tone, *'nice weather for the time of year'*, makes a mockery of my situation. Self-recrimination envelops me. *I should have realised! He's saying I should have realised earlier! It's my fault the shock is so great.*

I am hugely aware of my lungs; of the mechanics needed to be able to speak. Precious little air is coming in, but it's going out so fast there is none left for forming words. My body has seized up. It takes a huge effort to speak.

Bizarrely, I hear myself whisper agreement, while inside I'm shouting "No! No! *You said . . . you all said it was nothing to worry about. All the way along . . . 'nothing to worry about'. What a fool – I believed you! . . . My GP had laughed . . . she really hadn't known . . .*"

Why am I pretending I knew? I don't lie. What's happened to me? Is this what's meant by 'diminished responsibility' – like a person admitting to a crime they haven't committed? Perhaps I can't admit to being such a gullible fool. But that's what I am.

I've been taken in by con-men. They must have seen and felt the tumour when they first examined me, then again under anaesthetic, but there had been no hint. Nurses, doctors – so many people, would have known. Not me – yet it's my body. Why didn't they share their concerns from the outset? Why are they treating me like a child? Do I seem dim-witted?

He's talking again, his words fighting their way through porridge. With my senses painfully fired up to explode, I strain to process information, but thoughts whizz off at tangents. Concentrating with the intensity of a tightrope walker, I struggle to catch up, simultaneously logging, sifting, seeking comprehension. *How can this be? Keep control. Mustn't let the side down.*

"There are three options for treatment," he continues. "We can remove just the lump . . ." *Yes – great – go for it.* ". . . or we can remove a section of bowel and give you a colostomy . . ." *A bag? Horror of horrors!* ". . . or you can have radiotherapy." Fear of the unknown grips me. I am barely breathing now.

"The first option is the most likely, since it has not invaded the muscle," he slips in, easily.

'Since it has not invaded the muscle'! I had not thought about it invading any muscle. But that's good. It's just a little lump. Easy to take out. I hang onto that thought.

"We'll make an appointment with the oncologist in two days' time to discuss treatment." *What's an oncologist?*

The interview is coming to an end. But I need to know if I have any chance! From somewhere, a voice croaks, "What are my chances?"

"Very good. You are young . . ." *No I'm not. I'm nearly fifty-one. And what has age got to do with it?* ". . . and the survival rate is 75–80%."

He seems relieved to be talking about this. Noticeably more relaxed.

No word of comfort. No hand in mine. No written information. No sources of support. I leave clutching an appointment card. I have cancer and I might die. I am to have treatment of some sort, but I don't know when. *And I might die.* There is no-one I can tell. *And soon, I might be dead.* How long do I have . . .? Cancer patients get told how long they've got, don't they? Why haven't they told me? I feel cheated.

I emerge from the hospital in a drunken daze. My brain has been replaced by a mass of tightly knotted wire linked to an explosive device and count-down has begun. People walk past me. Traffic is flowing. A bird sings. The world around me continues to function as if nothing has happened.

Somehow, I totter to the car and drive home.

DISCUSSION

How did it feel when the consultant ignored you?
It felt like a discourteous demonstration of his authority.

Why do you think this happened?
He had not read my case notes in preparation for the consultation and was catching up.

What did you think of the manner of delivery?
It felt cruel. He seemed determined to retain a pretence of normality at any price, to prevent having to deal with my emotions.

What effect did this have on you?
The lack of openness, coupled with brutal delivery, damaged my trust in the medical profession, at a time when I most needed it and with long-term consequences.

Why do you think he asked if you thought you had a tumour?
I felt it allowed him to pretend I had been prepared – that he had not caused me harm. If he had been checking my understanding, it was cruelly inappropriate timing because of what had gone before.

How did it make you feel?
Doubly humiliated.

Were you able to remember what was said to you after being given the diagnosis?
Every word, every part of the consultation, kept replaying in my head.

What needed to change?
Doctors need to familiarise themselves with case notes in advance of consultations.

Clinicians delivering bad news need specific training,[3] or they are likely to cause harm and affect a patient's subsequent adjustment.[4]

The benefits of taping significant consultations are now well recognised.[5,6] Patients can check and come to terms with what has been said and formulate questions, saving time at the next consultation.

I needed:
» complete honesty and openness
» to be advised from the outset that cancer was a distinct possibility
» to be encouraged, *with emphasis*, to bring someone to consultations
» to be asked how much I wanted to know
» to be put in touch with a cancer nurse specialist
» to be given a tape of the consultation
» to be enabled to communicate my needs and feelings
» privacy, support and time to recover
» to be put in touch with other people who had the same cancer.

I needed written information on:
» my particular type of cancer
» treatment options
» local and national cancer charities and support groups (including independent groups)
» state benefits.

Chapter 5 ▪

Credit me
Pinch my cheeks
And rub in lipstick
Buff the sparkle in my eyes
Fix the smile and stretch the backbone
Then I'll get straight information
Instead of porky pies

That evening, as I walk the dogs through our fields before heading down the lane, I take a hard look at my surroundings, remembering the day we moved in. Ancient oaks nestle among overgrown hedgerows tumbled with honeysuckle, their grassy banks strewn with wild flowers. A small orchard of gnarled but productive apple trees lies squeezed between the fields and beyond that a fruit and vegetable patch, a sanctuary where hundreds of birds rear their young each year. Swallows and house martins, attracted by rich pickings, swoop over the muck-heap and, as evening falls, fluttering bats take their place.

It has been my sanctuary too, a place to lose myself in the beauty of nature. Living in a relationship that has irretrievably broken down can be extremely stressful. I feel trapped. We no longer communicate, except out of necessity, playing 'happy families' if society demands. When my friends call, there is a veneer of normality, like thinly spread jam: too earnest, unconvincing. The stress is grinding us both down. Life has become an endurance test. We do not entertain and have no shared social life.

Being able to get away to riding events has made life bearable. But always, on the return journey, an inevitable air of gloom overlays any elation, like a cloudburst about to wreck a picnic. It has become routine to concentrate hard on the road and hope my daughter will not notice my brimming eyes. Now, that life has become incredibly precious.

I don't feel ill – how can I have cancer? *I don't feel ill*! I'm the one who writes the prescriptions and dispenses the medicines. I don't take pills, except for HRT (hormone replacement therapy). I'm one of the healthy ones. Even when I have 'flu, I battle on in disbelief until I can't lift the kettle.

What do I know about cancer? I've heard cancer patients have someone assigned to support them, one to one, throughout treatment, but I haven't got anyone. I wonder when they'll contact me. A frantic memory-trawl dredges up glimpses of childhood as I recall the gravely voices of two ashen-faced neighbours who'd died from lung cancer. They stank like wet ashtrays. Children notice these things.

In our small village there's a farmer with lung cancer. Another, with bowel cancer, sits for hours on the village green (waiting to die?). There used to be a yellowy-grey woman, too. Maybe she's dead. Does chemotherapy sap your colour? I'll never be yellow. I'll rub lipstick into my cheeks. Another man, just outside the village, gets taken off in one of those rattling 'sit up and beg' mini-bus ambulances – known to patients as 'cattle-trucks' – day after day. "He's terminal, but he doesn't know it," the GP had confided to me one day. I'd thought it dreadfully wrong that I knew, but he didn't. *Are they keeping the truth from me?*

So many people in one small hamlet. What else? I've read about Bob Champion, the jockey who overcame cancer, then won a race. But what I remember most are his months of vomiting and that friends remarked on his grumpiness. *I won't change!* But how will I cope with months of being sick?

An old TV series about a man given six months to live, who travelled America doing good deeds, had seemed romantic at the time, but he was only acting. *How long do I have? Should I be travelling the world, doing the things I've always longed to do?*

I need to share this with someone, but there is no-one. I'll tell my husband once treatment has been decided, when the practicalities need working out. The children don't need to know yet. I'll protect them as long as possible. Can't tell close friends, or they'll suffer. That night I sleep little.

The waiting chasm had been well camouflaged by snow. I teeter for a moment,

scrabbling for hope, but the boot in the back catapults me into space and I'm

plummeting through inky blackness . . .

Next morning, I write prescriptions and hand out pills like an automaton. Later I'll wonder how many people were given the wrong medicines that day. Kath, my co-receptionist is her usual bouncy self. We get on well and share the admin jobs in this small practice, making appointments, writing repeat prescriptions, ordering, dispensing and even delivering medicines to elderly or house-bound people. I also type a few letters and sometimes fill in as baby-sitter for the doctor's children and I'm in line to train as Practice Manager, not that I want to make a career of this job. Our wages are low, but we recently had a small pay rise.

The morning drags on. My head is bursting, but I feel I must tell my GP first. She knows I changed my work rota to attend hospital the previous day and will be wondering how I got on. At last surgery is ending. I slip my head around the door.

"Can I see you for a minute?"

"Nope. Got to rush. It'll have to wait." She gathers up her things and rushes out.

It's the regular Tuesday GP meeting at the local hospital and attendance merits GP 'Brownie' points. Of course, she thinks I have anal warts, so I understand. All the same, I'm left suspended in a vacuum. No visible means of support.

Kath's humming a little tune. I feel sorry for her. I'm about to spoil her day.

"I went to the hospital yesterday," I begin.

"Oh yes. How did you get on?" she smiles, always ready with a joke. 'Ebullient', that's Kath. I love her cheery smile. We'd shared a few laughs about bottoms when I first mentioned my problem. Now the pot boils over. "It's not anal warts," I tell her. "I've got cancer."

Poor Kath. It's like grounding a kite. She looks so crestfallen, I wish I could take it back, but 'need to offload' overcomes guilt and I plough on, selfishly. Even more unfairly, I ask her not to tell anyone until I have told my family.

Chapter 6

Smiles are not enough

And now I'm passed from one to another
And find there is even more to discover
You don't seem to value the thing I most need
But without it, I bleed

I so much want to believe in your smile
But it's clicked on and off (to cover the guile?)
Why can't you see that, by shutting me out
You leave me in doubt

"Are you well?" The innocent Yorkshire greeting jolts me next day as I pay for petrol. *Actually, I've got cancer. I'm on my way to see an oncologist. Oh yes – and I'm going to die.* Dismissing such thoughts, I manage a faint nod and a wry smile and hurry outside.

My feet belong to someone else. Like Moira Shearer in 'The Red Shoes'[7] I'm being forced to walk where I don't want to go: through the hospital entrance – into the general waiting area – try not to meet anyone's eye. Have they all got cancer, too? Is there time to go to the loo? But my name rings out – the voice seems loud and strident. I cringe. Like dutiful schoolchildren, or mesmerised tourists, we follow in caterpillar squiggle to the next waiting area. *'Around this corner, ladies and gentlemen . . . and to your right, housed behind anonymous doors, are the Unapproachables, Guardians of the Unthinkables and Unmentionables' – and on your left, a collection of the Untouchables . . .'*

It's stressing me out just having to sit here. I perch, bolt upright, ears straining in readiness for my name to slice through the silence. And there's not long to wait. Multiple pairs of eyes follow my every movement as I stand on command to be ushered into the consulting room.

"I don't need to get undressed, I'm only here to discuss treatment"

I gabble. The nurse throws me a quizzical look, but smiles and says the doctor will be with me shortly, as she exits through a side door. I'm left alone. It probably isn't long before the oncologist (cancer doctor) comes in, but seconds are mimicking hours. My stomach feels like the interior of a golf ball. My bowels are practising knitting.

Smiles all round. After shaking my hand and introducing himself, he invites me to take a seat. And I hear myself say, "No, thanks. I'm OK."

Bizarre! Why don't I sit down? Do I think I can make a quick get-away? How foolish I must look! But still I remain standing. Putting on an act. *See? I can cope!*

Not surprisingly, he seems a little taken aback, but smiles equably and half sits on the examination bed, remarking, "Well, I'll take the weight off my feet anyway." The friendly, informal manner is immediately reassuring. The kind eyes and caring tone invite trust. I feel he will do his best to save my life.

"There are two options for treatment," he is saying, the voice as soft as summer rain, "Removing just the lump is not possible since it has invaded the muscle."

Two options? It *has* invaded the muscle? *No! That's wrong . . . he told me . . .* A flurry of icicles finds its target. I'm caught up in conflict: grateful for the gentle tone, yet unable to accept the dispar-ity of this distorted echo of the first consultant's words.

There have been no further investigations . . . *so there never had been a third option!*

The first doctor had known all along and lied! *Stupid! Stupid! Stupid!* I'm curling up in humiliation, struggling to get to grips with this. Yet again, the double sledge-hammer: bad news compounded by deceit as shocking as my reduced options and as devastating as the cancer diagnosis itself. *Why should they equate 'patient' with 'child'? Why assume an authority over information about my body? Why, so cruelly raise false hopes?*

Self esteem plummets. I've been categorised, down-graded. Insecurity has reached critical phase. Don't they realise what lying and withholding information does to people? They are the only thing between me and death. I desperately need to be able to trust them, or I have nothing to rely on. But how can I trust them if they are not 100% honest with me?

"We can't remove all the tumour or the muscle would not work properly. You would need a colostomy – and you wouldn't want that."

He's telling me the tumour is in the anal canal, but has spread down into the muscle as well as along to the anus. Surgery would leave me with no control over my bowel movements. His voice is 'trust-me-kind', but the word 'colostomy' hangs between us, to be joined by 'chemotherapy . . . radiotherapy . . . radioactive implants' and side effects of 'nausea, diarrhoea, tiredness and wind'. *That doesn't sound too bad. What will all this mean? What do I need to ask?* Just when I need my brain to display some brilliant intellectual capacity, it's become a redundant computer, running on soup.

"Any questions?" – *(smile)*

I am still cowed by the deceit but, half prepared this time, pull a crumpled list from my pocket. It's difficult to speak without any air in your lungs and your stomach fused to your backbone. I focus hard on deciphering my scrawl and manage, "Will I be able to drive?"

"Yes."

There had been the slightest hesitation, but I pretend not to notice. It's so important to be able to retain my independence. *Not to have to be driven by my husband.* If there is a chance, I'll manage.

"Will I be incontinent?" – the dreaded word forced out in a barely audible whisper, despite the effort to make it sound like an everyday question.

There's an even more noticeable hesitation before, with supreme nonchalance, he returns, "Which – urinary or faecal?"

Red alert! He's playing for time. *Why suggest 'urinary' when the cancer's in my backside? Might I be doubly incontinent?* Thoroughly disconcerted, my senses are sucking in signals like giant antennae, my insides liquefying in dread.

"Both – either." I'm a high tension wire, ready to snap.

"Shouldn't be." – *(smile)*

'Shouldn't be'? Is that meant to reassure? If neither possibility is likely, why the prevarication? Sounds like fence-sitting to me. But I can't push.

"Will I lose my hair?"

"Only your pubic hair."

Hah! Never thought of that. Now a callow teenager, fighting to suppress a smirk, I press on with my list.

"What causes it?"

"We don't know."

"What's it called?"

"Squamous carcinoma of the anal canal."

"How big is it?"

"Four centimetres."

I'm still struggling to push out the words. I want to know what it looks like (must I fight imagined monsters?) and how the treatment works, but he has other patients and the nurse is saying, "So if you'd

24

like to slip off your clothes below the waist . . ." He's expecting to examine me!

They are both staring at me. I'm such a fool! Overcome with embarrassment for having misunderstood, but also at having to get undressed in front of an audience, I expect him to leave the room, or at least turn away. I'm not used to stripping naked in front of strangers. Just because they are health professionals does not make it any easier. Frozen in consternation, I look towards him expectantly. He seems rather amused, but turns away a little. Am I being ridiculous? In a few moments he is going to be looking at my naked body.[5]

Once I'm bare from the waist down, I lie rigidly, my eyes riveted on his face, ready to pick up the slightest signal.

"Just relax", he smiles encouragingly as he prods my abdomen, now tauter than a trampoline. But, as he fingers the lump in my groin, I watch the shutters come down. Seriousness hangs in the air. A frosted vice grips my insides.

"That's just a hern . . ." The distant, rasping voice drops away. Even before he answers, 'Who told you that?' I *know*. It's not a hernia. It never was a hernia. My GP had been wrong. The first consultant had intentionally misled me – twice. Cancer has spread to my lymph glands. *No chance now! I am going to die.*

"It's-in-the-lymph-isn't-it?" I seem to be using my in-breath to speak. There is precious little air passing either way.

"We don't know yet."

But I do. Why can't he just admit it? How long do I have, weeks? – Days?

I need him to talk about this. But there is no discussion. *('Don't worry your head about it – our problem'.)*

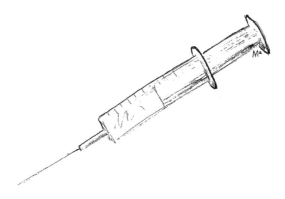

Figure 6.1 Help!

Dazed into horror-struck silence, I watch the nurse prepare a horse-sized needle. *I am going to be spiked to the bed, like a butterfly. They can't expect me to lie here while they stick that into my groin!* I want someone to hold my hand. I want to get up and run. *How much will it hurt?* But there's no reassurance. The silence intensifies.

I look away as the needle goes in and he draws fluid from the lump. It isn't very painful after all, but this fearsome procedure, on top of mounting deceit and multiple shocks, is just too much. A tear has collected in the corner of one eye. *Funny that, just the one eye.*

My mind is in overdrive, trying to find reason where there is none; to comprehend the incomprehensible.

Beyond the sausage skin
Disregard my wobbly lip
Ignore these foolish tears
Look beyond the quivering wreck
And credit me with at least a speck
Of the mettle I had before

With stainless steel my jaw is set
And my backbone may surprise you yet
With its carbon fibre core

I can get dressed. He's explaining about treatment. I'm to have a week in hospital, then radiotherapy as an outpatient. I have no idea what radiotherapy is, or what it entails. Radioactive implants. *What are they?* It's all a blur. I have no idea how long it will all take. Now they are asking me questions. I can't find words quickly enough. I feel like reinforced jelly. Breathing is so difficult. My mouth's not working properly. Can't they see I'm desperately in need of privacy and comfort? I feel like a prisoner under interrogation.

"I expect you are thinking, 'Why me?'"

Why should I be thinking that?

"No, I'm not! I've seen too many!" I have to hand over control of my body, but now they're making assumptions about the only thing I have left – my mind.

"What does your husband do?"

What has that to do with anything? It's so hard to speak.

"He's a poultry consultant," I blurt out. At least, that's what my head wants my mouth to say, but it's being uncooperative.

Stifled explosions of laughter grate incongruously in the highly charged atmosphere. They must have thought I said, 'paltry'

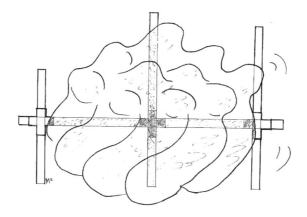

Figure 6.2 Reinforced jelly.

consultant! Damn! Why didn't I say 'agricultural' consultant . . .?
I want them to know I'm sharing the joke with them. *Look – I've
still got my sense of humour. See how strong I am!'* But my face
doesn't move a muscle. It's as if I'm semi-paralysed. The moment
passes. Opportunity lost.

*Why are they asking about neighbours? Will I need nursing?
Do they expect neighbours to get involved?* It's a small, northern
farming community. I'm a 'Southerner', an 'Outsider'. My closest
friends live miles away.

"Have you any children?"

I've held out until this point, but they have catapulted me into
thinking about the effect on my children.

"Four . . ." I bleat, but it's too much. I choke up. The nurse hands
me a tissue but it remains untouched in my lap. There are so many
questions I want to ask, but I can't speak. I can't bear the penetrating
eyes assessing 'how I am taking it'. My gaze drops to the floor. I'm
desperate to be alone, to think about what all this means.

"Sorry."

Why am I saying 'sorry'? *Must be brave, must be strong.* Don't
want them being too kind to me or I will crack up. They want me
to wait at the hospital until the sample has been tested, but I tell
them I'm already late for the school run.

"What's the 'school run'?"

Bemused, I manage only a dismembered staccato.

"Son . . . collect . . . school".

"Which school?"

What does it matter!

The tightness in my head is unbearable. *Stupid, not to have*

27

swapped places on the rota ... hadn't wanted anyone to know ... why don't they let me go ... children will be wondering where I am ...

The oncologist asks me to ring his direct number for results as soon as I'm home, then they'll organise treatment. But I have to drop neighbour's children first – it will be past five o'clock.

"Will you still be here?" I ask doubtfully, surprised when he nods.

I'm ashamed to have shown any weakness and want to let him know he needn't put on that sympathetic voice, but my mouth seems to have become disconnected from my brain. From now on, everything I say is passed through a garbelizer.

"I need you to talk to me in a 'matter of fact' tone of voice," I blurt incoherently, as I stand to leave and, in a last ditch attempt to get them to credit me, I add, "I may have a wobbly lip, but I can take it." This strange protestation brings a placatory smile – and probably just confirms their low opinion of me.

I can deal with bad news. I need them to respect me and not withhold information in future. I need to know everything. Everything!

The nurse sits me in the busy corridor alongside the patients' waiting area, while she gets his telephone number. I need privacy, yet I'm on public view. Deep in shock, I struggle to retain composure, breathe normally. Every mounting second is mega-stress. *I'm going to die ... children waiting ... try to keep face set at 'normal' – eyes down to hide the death sentence from curious strangers.*

The consultation replays over and over in my head. How on earth am I going to tell the family? How will I manage to drive home?

"Would you like a cup of tea?"

Hysteria threatens! So they really do give cups of tea to people who are going to die.

"No ..." The brief reply is all I can manage with semi-paralysed lungs. *Hope they'll understand. People will guess why she was offering tea ... hope nobody heard ... I don't drink tea!*

The nurse pops her head round the door, looks at me and bobs back again. Why didn't she bring that number? Did they sit me here just to monitor me? This is unbearable ... have to go ... so much kinder to let me go ... stress is off the scale ...

Just as I'm on the point of escaping, the nurse appears again and hands me a card. At last! Past a blur of faces – out of the double doors. Somehow, my legs get me to the car.

DISCUSSION

How did it feel to learn option 3 had never existed and the lump was not a hernia?

It was degrading to find I was not in their confidence and devastating to realise I could not trust them.

Wasn't it better to hear bad news in small doses and come to terms with it slowly?
No. It meant I had to deal with the consequences of deception, as well as with the diagnosis. There is no such thing as partial honesty.

Did the reply about lymph node involvement satisfy you?
No. I did not want meaningless reassurance. It must have been obvious from the way my voice dried that I realised the implications. I learned later that most patients with this cancer had inguinal node involvement at diagnosis.

Why didn't you ask how long you might survive?
Communication was doctor-led. I was in shock and passively expected them to tell me everything there was to know. Evasiveness blocked discussion. The mention of death (their failure?) seemed taboo.

How did it feel when they assumed you were thinking 'why me'?
It was unnerving to have those in control wrongly assume they knew what I was thinking. It felt as if their view of me would always be shaped by preconceptions – misconceptions. It was like being caught up in 'One Flew Over the Cuckoo's Nest',[8] a feeling continually reinforced during my cancer experience.

You were upset when they asked if you had any children?
The thought of causing my children to suffer was the worst aspect of diagnosis. The mother lion was about to harm her cubs. I needed to come to terms with this in my own time.

Why do you think they asked this question?
Naively, I reasoned it must be part of a routine way of helping people deal with the stress by prompting tears! It was inconceivable that such a hurtful question could be asked mindlessly.

Did lowering your eyes indicate you could not cope with more information?
Absolutely not! I wanted to know everything, but needed to hide my emotions.

What effect did their questioning have?
Being questioned, when trying to get to grips with the probability of dying, made things so much worse and felt unkind.

Did you feel you had been given a genuine choice of treatments?
Options were not discussed, although surgery was mentioned as a non-starter. I learned later that radiotherapy alone had been used successfully for some small anal cancer tumours.[9]

What was uppermost in your mind when you left the hospital?
I was terrified of having a road accident and killing the children.

You did not ask about support groups?
I'd never heard of support groups.

Do you think staff realised how shocked you were?
The letter to my GP said, 'she seemed stunned', as if my reaction had been surprising.

What needed to change?
Patients' understanding of their situation needs to be checked before treatment is discussed.

Use of decision aids can enable patients to express their information needs and treatment preferences.[10,11]

Staff communications skills training[12] could have prevented assumptions being made and facilitated more meaningful discussion.

I needed them to talk about the biopsy and what the results could mean.

I needed most of the same things I had needed when first given the diagnosis (see Chapter 4) and also:

» privacy for undressing and dressing
» full information on risks and benefits of treatment options
» full information on short and long term side effects, no matter how rare, in order to make an informed choice. Only I could know how these might affect my life.

Chapter 7

Overboard
Tangle of bodies, dropped en bloc
Threshing, flailing, clawing
Bobbing heads shouting, sinking
Cacophony!

And me
Stretching for the single rock in the empty, shore-less sea

Once again, I have no written information about my condition, treatments, or sources of help and no idea what information I might need or how to access it.

The traffic is heavy. When finally I reach them, the children stand in a huddle, cold wet and forlorn, like abandoned dogs. I mutter apologies, but can't offer an explanation of why I am late, or where I have been. Their puppy eyes deliver mute reproach as they clamber in. I'm full of self recrimination for having failed them and hope they'll chatter among themselves, avoid eye contact with me in the mirror, not read 'death' written there. But I needn't worry. They are tired, wet teenagers, their minds full of missed television programmes and evening homework. The air is heavy with disgruntled silence.

Concentrate on the road! Banish all thoughts of cancer, treatments, children, death, until I get home. How long before I can make that phone call? I need to know, now! Concentrate!

The windows soon steam up and darkness shelters me from prying eyes until we are forced to stop at a zebra crossing. I slump down, glad of the obscuring rain. As we join the notoriously dangerous dual carriageway, the rush hour is in full swing. I concentrate on the road with painful intensity. At last we reach the crossroads, just a mile from home, but I'm forced to turn in the opposite direction, then down an endless farm track, to drop off the first child. The rain is relentless. "Goodbye. Sorry I was late." Back to the infamous black spot crossroads. *Concentrate!* Into the village, drop off remaining children. Somehow we arrive home without fatalities.

The children give searching looks when I bustle them into the sitting room and ask them to stay there while I make a private phone call, but I can't explain. A protective barrier has sprung up between us. I can't even think about how I'm going to tell them. I have to concentrate on this call to the consultant, the focus of my hope. My head feels as if it will implode.

It's ringing. I wonder if he's still there. He answers. I give my name.

"I'm afraid the results show there are some cancer cells present . . ."

'Some'? In a lump the size of a pea there must be thousands! *Stop minimalising!*

So I'm going to die. I don't want to go through terrible treatment if it means my last few weeks will be ruined. *'He's terminal, but he doesn't know it'* . . . bounces around my brain. After so much deception, how can I trust them?

Struggling with paralysed lungs, I try to enunciate slowly, clearly and in capital letters (there must be no mistake about this), "PLEASE, TELL ME HONESTLY, DO I HAVE ANY CHANCE?"

My voice sounds pretty normal. I'm pleased about that. The whole situation is about as normal as walking willingly to execution and checking the blade of the guillotine.

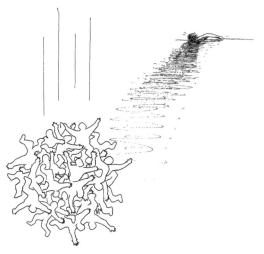

Figure 7.1 Overboard.

"Certainly. A very good chance."

His voice is normal, too. Not over-solicitous. Good. But I'm not convinced. When cancer spreads, people die. Everyone knows that. I don't want false hope. How can I believe him?

"So we'll go ahead with treatment?"

But I can't decide. I don't know enough. *Are you telling the truth?*

"That depends . . ."

"On what?"

"On how good a liar you are."

"Hrrmmph!" He chokes back his surprise.

I'm more surprised than him. I don't talk to doctors like that! I don't talk to *anyone* like that! And I don't mean to be rude, I'm simply desperate for honesty. It's as if I've taken a truth drug – all the social niceties have been stripped away. *We are down to bare essentials here.* Nothing matters except that he is honest with me.

He says they wouldn't be going to all this trouble if I didn't have a chance. I want to believe him. I need to believe *in* him. *He is going to save my life.* Without much difficulty, I let myself be persuaded. Treatment will begin in about two weeks' time.

I replace the receiver like a sleepwalker and call the children for refreshments. My legs are jelly. My head's in a vice. Thankfully, I'm left alone as my daughter goes outside to bring in the horses and bed them down, while my son watches TV before doing his homework. No questions yet. I long for bed, to be alone, to have time to think. There is a meal to prepare, chickens to be fed and shut up for the night. I take the dogs with me. Always glad of the chance to let off steam, they run helter-skelter after rabbits, real and imaginary, tongues lolling. There is something comforting, if poignant, about their innocent play. Wet noses nudge my hand. Unconditional love. How strange to think they may be chasing rabbits this time next year without me.

Two weeks is a long time. Why wait to begin treatment? The cancer will be growing and spreading every minute! They are just pretending I have a chance or they would be starting it now.

I go through the motions of making supper. I can't eat. It's like forcing down dry cardboard. Thankfully, nobody notices. We don't eat together at the table like a normal family, except when it's unavoidable. No-one can bear the forced conversations, the silences.

Now I'm playing another role, living yet another pretence.

The evening drags on, but eventually I can creep to bed and lick my wounds. Sleep is out of the question. I spend that whole night, and the next, writing 'good-bye' letters to my children. It's difficult to write an individual message to each of them. Repetition diminishes sincerity. How can I convey how much I love them? What pearls of wisdom should I be passing on? To my husband I write something about us 'growing apart'. He must not feel any guilt. It takes two . . . and it's important that no-one has bad memories of me when I am gone. I cannot leave a legacy of hurt. I put them in an envelope marked, 'To be opened in the event of my death'.

DISCUSSION

Wasn't it reasonable to say there were 'some' cancer cells present?
Yes, my reaction was 'over the top'.

Why was it 'over the top'?
I was in shock, so my senses were fully charged, my reactions exaggerated. Because they had lied, I was now over-analytical, trying to sift truth from fiction.

Did you want to be given biopsy results over the phone?
Yes, absolutely! Every second of not knowing was worse than the worst news. I was very grateful.

You gave your consent to treatment over the telephone?
Things were different in those days. Apparently, I signed a form later, for the implant procedure. It was standard procedure because of risks associated with general anaesthesia. I knew of no other risks. There was no consent 'process'.

Giving properly informed consent for radical or invasive procedures should now be an audited process, not just a case of 'getting a signature'.[13]

Patients need full information about treatments, risks and benefits if they are to give informed consent.

Chapter 8

I've come to work as usual but it's been impossible to concentrate. This time, my GP does have time to see me. Sitting at her desk like a real patient, I begin with difficulty, "I saw the consultant . . ."

"Oh yes. How did you get on?" she cuts in brightly. So she hasn't heard the news yet.

I try to carry on speaking but I'm choked up. I've had very little food or sleep for four days now. All this time, a sledgehammer has been beating at my skull and a guillotine, fastened to cotton thread, has been poised above my head.

"Come on! It can't be that bad!" she laughs.

Fighting to keep control, I force the words out in a single whoosh. "I've got cancer and it's spread and I've got to have radiotherapy and chemotherapy . . ." and choke to a stop.

'The smile was wiped from her face' – there it is again – only this time I see it happening on someone else. I have never seen anyone look so shocked. She sits gripped in disbelief, her jaw literally dropping open.

"I can't believe it . . . I can't believe it," she keeps muttering as she stares into space.

I wait expectantly, craving solace as the silence lengthens, but have to prompt gently, "It's not that easy for me . . ."

"I can't believe it," she repeats again, adding, "I only referred you because you work for me. If it had been anyone else, I'd have told them to go home and see how it went for a few weeks . . ."

Silence. I'm facing unknown horrors and I'm more than a little in need of comfort.

"I'm very frightened," I whisper. It's the first time I've allowed myself to think about fear, let alone voice it. And the tears win.

My words tilt her out of her trance. She gets up from the desk and puts an arm round my shoulders.

"If it gets too bad, will you end it for me?" I ask naively, and of course she agrees. But I'm not so sure she would. Her predecessor had told me about a friend with lung cancer who 'didn't think she could stand the pain much longer', yet took two more painful months to die. If doctors can't control their friends' pain, what chance do others have? I've heard some doctors under-prescribe morphine for fear of being blamed for patients' deaths. Surely, if a patient needs better pain control, they should have it, whether or not it shortens life? I'm beginning to wish I were a dog.

When I emphasize my need for complete honesty, however bad the news, she promises to be straight with me. She's surprised treatment won't start for another two weeks and I tell her I wish it could be sooner. My head is tight with emotional turmoil and competing practicalities. How will Kath manage? Who will replace me here at such short notice?

"I don't know how I'm going to be able to afford to keep the horses."

"Don't worry," she reassures me, "You can have full pay for six months and we'll review things after that."

That's a great weight off my mind. My husband is currently out of work. She suggests I go home. I suppose it is strange to keep working when I may be 'time limited'. After exchanging hugs with Kath, I leave, relief edged with truant's guilt. No longer 'staff', I'm just a patient – truly on the other side of the fence.

What needs to be done? What do I need for hospital? I don't own a decent nightdress. Money! Is there enough food in the freezer? Might be ill for months . . . might die . . . contingency plans. Daughter will have to learn how to tow the trailer this weekend. How will she manage to load the horse by herself? Car insurance. Have to tell the children. Need to make a will. I'm going to die. Am I going to die?

DISCUSSION

How did it feel to be breaking bad news to your GP?
It felt peculiar.

Did you think all cancer patients suffered pain?
I thought they had painful deaths. I knew of several whose pain had not been adequately controlled.

What needed to change?
» GPs should receive same-day notification when a patient is diagnosed with cancer.
» GPs' communication skills should enable patients to express their greatest fears and to deal competently with their replies.[12]

- » The medical curriculum should include more training in pain relief.
- » Some palliative care training should be mandatory for all GPs.
- » Increased numbers of specialists in palliative care are needed.[14]

Chapter 9

I've told my husband the news, but didn't register his reaction. Now I must tell my daughter. I try to come at things from another angle. Gently.

"I'm not going to be able to drive for a while. You will need to learn to tow the horse-box. We'll have to put you on the insurance." Rapid-fire short sentences sputter out.

She gives me a hard look. "Why?"

"I've got to go into hospital *'I've got to go into hospital' – I still can't believe this is happening.*

"For how long?" she asks, the hard look becoming an anxious, penetrating stare.

"I don't know."

I can't meet her eyes. I'm functioning like a decrepit robot and don't know how to soften the blow.

"I'm afraid I've got cancer." *Plop!* There it is. Lack of food and sleep no mitigation for the clumsy delivery. And I've just remembered – her college friend's mother recently died of cancer. As she moves away and opens the stable door *(for privacy – to have a cry?)* I'm wondering frantically how to protect her. Desperate to conjure some semblance of normality, I blurt out, "We all have to go some day." I have accepted the probability of death and now, somewhat insanely, seem to be trying to pretend it's no big deal! Drowning in inadequacy, I scrabble to make things easier for her and add, "No-one lives forever" – *as if that will make it acceptable!* I've just added a block of cement to a ton of bricks.

She starts to cry. I flounder on, "It's OK. I'm going to beat it." *Yeah, right!* But it's too late.

The children have to be able to carry on without me, so I'm trying to make light of things, but whatever I say is making things worse for her. I would die for her, yet I am hurting her. Frustration mixes with guilt. When I tell her brother, I make it brief and get a 'manly' phlegmatic response.

That evening, I telephone my two older sons. Both will have a five hour drive to visit me. I hate to be a nuisance. One by one, I lay the 'bad news' groundwork. I'm getting better at this. When I suggest they might like to sit down, amused disbelief gives way to nervous apprehension. Despite the distance, their shock is palpable. It's like sticking needles into them. I wish I could give them a hug. When they ask about my chances, instinctively, I say I don't know. That's another lie. I'm behaving out of character to protect them. Better that no-one knows what I know.

Kath visits later and brings a typed note from my GP requesting the return of the surgery key for my replacement and announcing I'll be on full pay for 3 months, rather than 6. She will review things after that.

The next few days are spent trailing around town in search of decent nightclothes. Nightgown or pyjamas? A mountainous decision. Days later, I buy pyjamas and instantly wonder if I've done the right thing. Car insurance is arranged and on Sunday I accompany my daughter as she drives car and trailer to her riding lesson.

"Hallo – how are you?"

Although anticipated, the trainer's greeting knots my stomach.

"Fine."

This might be the last time I see you, the last time I watch my daughter ride here.

The hour passes too quickly. As we prepare to leave, my 'goodbyes' are tinged with special regret. "See you next month", he says, cheerfully unaware.

With tricky manoeuvring, my daughter successfully aligns the trailer alongside a building at the first attempt, so the horse is encouraged to walk up the ramp – and he goes straight in! My daughter's better at this than I am!

DISCUSSION

Why did you withhold information from your family?
I had the right to protect my children. (The clinicians had no such right over me. They simply assumed a position of authority.)

How did you feel when you were told 6 months' pay was no longer guaranteed?
I felt written off.

Why did your boss change her mind about your pay?
Apparently, the Family Practitioner Committee (FPC) could not guarantee

to fully reimburse her for longer than 3 months. Later, I discovered they had never refused 6 months' full pay to anyone in this position.

Chapter 10

Eating and sleeping have become things of the past. Nothing matters except survival, for the children's sakes. The thought of making a will had flitted through my mind occasionally in the past, but was something to do when I became old. Now I may not grow old. Explaining to the solicitor's secretary why I need an urgent appointment is stressful. Climbing the stairs to their office is worse. I am about to make vital decisions which will affect my children within the context of my death. And my head is a wasps' nest of chewed paper.

The process is eased by a softly spoken lady solicitor who swiftly and expertly unravels my knotted thoughts. We part without realising for what purpose I will be engaging her services again.

Diarrhoea and insomnia are draining me. I feel increasingly unwell and have to lie down each afternoon. If they wait much longer there won't be anything left of me to treat. When my GP phones and suggests she could try to get treatment started earlier, I'm grateful and ask her to tell the oncologist I want to know everything. He will listen to her. Later that day she phones to say I'm being admitted in three days' time. It's frightening, but such a relief to know the fight is about to begin. She asks me to call and see her.

"It's very *unusual*, Mitzi," she says of the cancer, smiling tentatively, as if its very rarity should somehow make this killer disease more acceptable. *Playing things down? Self-justification?* Either way, I'm not blaming her for not recognising cancer. Trust me to get the unusual one.

I remember hearing that cancer feeds on hormones and she agrees I should stop taking HRT. She offers sleeping pills, but I don't want to take strong drugs, so she gives me a sample of something mild left by a drugs representative.

"Do you know what my chances are, now that it's spread to the lymph nodes?" I ask.

Is there any chance, or are they are stringing me along?

"Apparently, your chances have dropped to fifty-fifty."

The impact of bad news is overridden by gratitude for her honesty. Someone is not afraid to tell me the worst. *And I'll make sure I choose the right fifty.*

"It's very *unusual*, Mitzi . . ."

DISCUSSION

You were not angry that your GP had not recognised cancer?
No. I felt quite sorry for her, especially when I learned how little cancer training GPs were given and how few cases they saw each year.

Your consultant did not tell you to discontinue HRT?
No. Later I learned that anal cancer does not feed on hormones and if I had continued to take HRT it would probably have alleviated the side effects of treatment.

How did that make you feel?
Unnecessary suffering is hard to accept.

What needed to change?
Doctors involved in cancer care need to communicate fully with each other so that information does not conflict.

Interdisciplinary education could strengthen partnerships and improve communication in multidisciplinary teams and between primary, secondary and tertiary care.

Chapter 11 ▬

A friend drives me to the hospital, which is about forty-five miles away. She says the nurses there are hand-picked. That's encouraging. My departure had felt unreal, the 'goodbye's kept brief, for the children's sakes. "I'll be back" – a quick hug, a forced smile, eyes straining trying to look as if I believed it. *Wish I could think of something original to say. What if . . .? Will I ever see you again?*

An hour or so later I'm waving my friend off at the hospital entrance, impatient to get started. The adventurer in me welcomes the chance to show what I'm made of; the wimp wants to turn and run. 'Visceral' partly describes the churning in my guts, but what words could adequately convey this mixture of fear, hope, helplessness and threatened independence? It's much worse than the first day at school. I pull myself up tall and try to look confident, but my bulging bag signals 'new intake'. Might as well have a notice stuck to my forehead proclaiming, 'One of Them: Number 10,003.'

The hospital booklet said single rooms were available for a small charge, so it's an immense blow to learn these are all occupied. Of course I'm sorry for people who are really ill, but dealing with my own cancer is going to be quite enough, without having to suffer for others.

A plastic hospital identification 'bracelet' is fitted, my temperature and blood pressure checked. A nurse escorts me to have a blood sample taken, but when we arrive at the haematology department she is called away. As I sit alone in the corridor, a man in a white coat appears, sits down next to me and asks why I'm in hospital. When I tell him, he grabs my hand and encases it in two warm, comforting paws. (*I'm here. Everything's going to be all right.*)

"It's OK, I'm not nervous," I smile. But the feeble remonstration lacks conviction. And I leave my hand there.

"That's all right," he replies, "I'm enjoying it!"

We both laugh and I wonder if this is all part of the service. It feels so good. Yes, I'm 'Miss Independent', I can cope, but this human contact is giving me extra strength. And I do so need a hand in mine.

"Just a little scratch", they say as they take the blood sample, not that a needle piercing flesh bears any resemblance to a scratch. Then it's back to the ward and down to the serious business of being a cancer patient. I am keen to comply with the rules. If I have to be a patient, I'll be the best they've ever had.

A central passage runs the length of the ward which is partitioned into two sections, each containing 8 beds with individual TV sets. I'm pleased to find my bed is in a corner, next to a window. My small corner. I set about home-making, covering the locker with photos of my children, tapes and tape recorder, and the armchair next to it with books. They've told me I can get undressed and into bed, but I'm not ill so I change into nightclothes, sit on the top cover and began to take stock.

It's freezing. Expecting a hot-house environment, I've brought only a thin summer housecoat. The large window is open just a crack, but it's enough for a chilly wind to find its way in. Despite the discomfort, the fresh air is an unexpected bonus, cutting through the alien hospital atmosphere and bringing with it a taste of freedom. I cherish it like a starving prisoner guards a morsel of cheese, pull the bedcover over my legs and hope no-one will notice and close the window.

I'd imagined the place would be bursting at the seams, but the adjoining bed is empty. There are two women across from me; one, directly opposite, is elderly and, I realise, very ill. *Will I be like that soon?* There are four more patients across the middle division, but I can only glance perfunctorily at them.

I am in a cancer hospital. I did not know such places existed. It feels as if I have been plucked from society and dropped into a leper colony.

Soon, a nurse comes and fits a cannula into my arm. "Have you had one before?" she asks. *Is she so used to cancer recurring?* I tell her I'm a first-timer. She explains it's similar to having blood taken. I hardly feel a thing. Her voice is kind. Her smile is caring. I feel in safe hands.

Pretty soon I'm attached to a 'lamppost' contraption with two bags of fluid suspended from it and a pump making rhythmical 'chukka-chukka' noises. Every now and again it goes a little crazy and chatters haphazardly out of sinc. Jazz! Great! Labels show I'm having a mixture of Fluorouracil (5FU) and Mitomycin C (MMC). There's also a bag of saline 'because your electrolytes are down'. *What are they?* I'm told to let the nurses know if anything becomes uncomfortable. *How bad is their 'uncomfortable'? What could go wrong? How quickly could they turn off the pump . . .?*

The fluids flood into my body. Hurrah! They're killing the cancer! It's so good to know the fight has begun, although I'm nervous about what the drugs might do to me. Once I'm sure chemotherapy doesn't hurt, it's fascinating to listen to the pump chuntering away and I fall deeper into the role of 'cancer patient', putting my life into the hands of strangers with blind faith.

The lamppost has wheels, so I can be mobile. Great! Moving gingerly at first, in case I pull the cannula, I set off to investigate the toilets. They are just around the corner opposite the nurses' station (*poor nurses!*), but still quite a distance if I have urgent need and I've had diarrhoea since being diagnosed. The open door reveals a row of basins facing a row of lavatories. *No privacy for washing. How will I cope with diarrhoea? What if I'm sick simultaneously? How will I bear the sounds and smells when other people vomit?* Tucked away behind the door, I notice a single chair.

Back on the bed, I'm feeling less confident. But what's really gnawing away at me is growing despair at the thought of distressing my children. I need to get away from all these sick people, but nurses say a doctor is expected on the ward shortly.

It's not the oncologist, but a young doctor with a thoughtful face and a sincere smile. He asks his questions, listens with his stethoscope, does his doctor thing – but he does not ask to examine my bum!

"I expect you are fed up with people looking at your bottom," he says gently – and I want to hug him! How considerate! But I just give a little nod. It's still hard to talk. He's given me back a little dignity. I didn't catch his name, but I will never forget his face.

Shortly afterwards, a nurse escorts me downstairs for radiotherapy planning. *Why don't they tell me where to go and let me find my own way? Do some patients try to escape?* As I sit down, my 'guard's' bleep sounds and, apologising profusely, she hurries away, and it's only then that I realise how comforting it had been to have someone with me. What a contrary creature I am.

So I'm sitting here, alone, in yet another corridor, shivering with cold *(why is it so cold?)* and fear of the unknown, wondering where everyone has gone. The oncologist pops his head around a door and spots me. I try to look serenely confident and hope he won't notice the shivering. Is he coming to get me? No, he's disappeared again. *It's the waiting that's always so terrible, isn't it* A few minutes later a nurse appears and takes me into his room.

"How are you?" The soft voice oozes reassurance, the smile exudes supreme confidence.

"Fine."

The hospital environment is intimidating enough, but being in the presence of One-Who-Can-Save-My-Life is awesome and it's too difficult to hold contact with those penetrating eyes.

Time to get undressed and lie half naked again as I'm measured and my skin marked for radiotherapy planning. Going topless on the beach will be easy after this. I try to concentrate on a mark on the wall and count to ten while lying under a huge machine called a simulator as radiotherapy staff plan precise individual treatment. It's scary but there's no radiation this time. According to my GP, the oncologist is one of the best in the country. I'm so lucky. It's so important for me to have confidence in him. *You are going to save my life. I know you will do your best for me. But if things don't work out, you mustn't feel any guilt.*

Never before have I felt so completely dependent on one person. Never before have I felt so alone.

DISCUSSION

What made you feel like a prisoner?
I had to stay there, because my life depended on it. Contributing factors

were: limited and conflicting information and the sense of being controlled.

Why could you only glance at patients furthest from you?
It was hard enough to deal with my own and my immediate neighbours' illnesses.

You wanted independence, yet missed the nurse's presence?
Yes.

So sometimes there is no right or wrong way of doing something?
That's right. I suppose I was fighting against becoming dependent. It must be difficult to address people's different needs.

What needed to change?
There should be sufficient single rooms so that patients do not have to deal with other people's suffering as well as their own.

Chapter 12 ▬

Death Row?
Sixteen beds, but isolation
Heaving wards of shell-shocked faces
Overwhelmed by all the sadness
By the scale of desolation
By the role that staff must play

Chemotherapy lamppost pumping
In rude health, apart from cancer
Sit *upon* the bed, not in it
Just a vain and futile gesture
But it's something I can do
I'm the one who's going to beat it
I'm not ill. I'm not like you!
But they're dying all around me
Did they think the same way, too?

Simultaneous radiotherapy
And a *wheelchair* now appears
(Though I'm capable of walking)

Challenge, and permission's granted
But the seed is deeply planted
Now confirmed: my deepest fears

It's quite clear, what they're expecting
It's quite clear what is assumed
Shockingly, yet just routinely
Everybody thinks I'm doomed

'Essence of cabbage', reminiscent of school dinners, hits my stomach long before we get back to the ward. I can't bear to look at the food trolley. Whatever is for lunch, I know I won't be able to eat it. I've eaten little since the diagnosis almost two weeks ago, but I don't feel hungry. It doesn't matter. The nauseating smell drives me to seek fresh air. I wish there was a balcony. Time to go exploring.

"Can I go for a little walk?" I ask tentatively, the new girl not wanting to put a foot wrong.

They ask me not to go far because I'm due for radiotherapy this afternoon. Wheeling my lamppost with care, I break free. Away from all those beds, all those sick people and out into uncharted territory. Anonymous and pretending to be healthy, I become a person again. We get up speed and whizz past a 'Visitors' Room' and 'Patients' Sitting Room' and I'm just considering using the lamppost as a scooter, when a gaggle of visitors comes pouring round the corner, staring curiously as they approach. *Yes. You can look! I'm one of 'Them'.* Labelled by lamppost, I become a heroine, fighting death. But as they draw near, I look away. I don't want their eyes to reflect pity.

There won't be any visitors for me. I've asked friends and family not to visit, to spare them long journeys, stilted bedside conversations, upsetting sights – and perhaps dreadful last memories. I walk on against the tide of visitors, but eventually turn and shuffle back feeling weak, dizzy and nauseous. As I turn the corner, a hubbub spills into the corridor: the ward has become an explosion of noise as TV programmes and people's voices compete.

Hoping to counter one noise with another I slip completely under the bedclothes clutching a small radio, but even with a finger in one ear and the radio pressed against the other, it's impossible to blot out the racket. Suddenly, daylight floods in as a nurse pulls back the covers.

"I thought you had a wire sticking out of your head," she says, indicating the aerial, concern quickly turning to amusement. She checks there are no problems with my chemo-pump or cannula, and leaves.

The radio no longer holds any attraction. I just want peace and quiet. Suddenly, a man appears at my bedside with – horror of horrors – a wheelchair!

"I've come to take you down to radiotherapy," he says.

My stomach plummets. So I was right all along. They're expecting me to deteriorate quickly – death is imminent.

"Do I have to use . . . *that*?"

He looks perplexed and seeks advice from a nurse.

"What's the problem?"

"Do I have to go in . . . *that*?" I nod towards the tangible reminder of my impending disablement, fearful she will insist. "I can walk. There's nothing wrong with my legs." I'm gabbling now.

She seems surprised and says patients usually travel to radiotherapy by wheelchair, but yes, I can walk if I want to. Victory! *For how long?* We set off, blanket, shawl-like around my shoulders, lamppost whizzing along at arm's length like a keen terrier. I find myself walking faster and faster, perhaps trying to show the world that wheelchairs aren't for the likes of healthy me. When we pass the main entrance I see why it has been so cold. Maintenance work being carried out on the entrance doors allows a marauding wind to infiltrate the whole building, scooping remnants of warmth from the remotest corners. Somewhere in a maze of corridors, I'm passed onto radiotherapy staff. *Corridors . . . catacombs . . .* Now I understand why I need an escort. They leave me sitting with other patients. As a distraction from my frozen ankles, I examine the 'Thank you' cards decorating the wall. Survivors. *Will someone sit here looking at my card one day?*

After a short while I'm taken to sit on a chair immediately outside the radiotherapy room. There is no entrance door, just a curtain. A woman emerges. It's my turn.

I step through and find there's a chair for my clothes just the other side. As I disrobe, I'm acutely aware of the next patient, just a curtain away and of several people standing by a gigantic machine, all looking at me. I hadn't realised I'd have to become a stripper. It's a long walk from chair to machine.

The radiotherapy staff are incredibly meticulous, yet remarkably patient and considerate. They deal with a constant stream of people, yet seem to show a genuine interest in me.

"Will it hurt?" I ask nervously. *It's a very big machine.* They assure me I won't feel a thing. But are they telling the truth?

They leave the room while treatment is delivered and I put my confidence in them. *Together we will beat it!* They tell me it will only take a few minutes. All I have to do is lie still, breathe normally – and, presumably, try not to be embarrassed at being naked from the waist down! Although they can watch me and talk to me through an intercom, I feel totally vulnerable: a car on an automated production line, in the hands of a gigantic robot.

Radiotherapy is given to my whole pelvic area, from navel to beyond my groins, with more targeted treatment directed from behind. And they were right – I didn't feel a thing. *Hurrah! This is going to be easy!*

When I emerge through the curtain, there is a man sitting on the chair. On the way back, I notice changing-cubicles and wonder why they are not in use.

Tea-time brings relief from ward noise. The choice is wholemeal or brown bread sandwiches, but I've been told to avoid all roughage. When a nurse notices I haven't eaten anything she orders white bread, but none is available. I don't mind. Eating takes effort. Eating means nausea. People can survive for weeks on fluids. I've been told to drink plenty, but they didn't say why.

Visiting time is in full swing when a nurse brings a telephone to my bed. It's my daughter. She's being so brave and supportive and has taken my place on the school transport rota, as well as coping with the last year of a time-consuming Higher National Diploma fashion course. Reluctantly, I ask if her father will bring my thick dressing-gown.

It's a long day, but eventually lights are dimmed. But there's no real peace. The poor lady in the opposite bed is very ill and has fits of coughing. Well, it's not so much coughing as *trying* to cough. My chest tightens in sympathy. Her pathetic struggles break the silence repeatedly as I try to sleep. I want to keep strong to be able to fight cancer, but it's too light, the bed is rock-hard and whenever I'm close to floating off the coughing starts again. Night closes in. Nurses patter to and fro. And I'm wide awake. *Drat! Now I need the loo! All this drinking . . .*

Adeptly gathering up my lamppost, I slide off the bed. The duty nurse asks if I am all right as I pass by. After trying to urinate as quietly as possible, I'm mortified when the flush cracks the night open in exaggerated crescendo.

Finally, aided by one of the sample sleeping pills, I drop off, only to be woken by squeaking and clattering as new oxygen cylinders are wheeled past. There is urgent whispering. Purposeful footsteps come and go. Everyone else seems to be asleep, but I lie here, sensing the crisis. Cough, cough, cough. My stomach knots up. I want to cough for her. *Is that how I will end?* I realise I'm lying in the foetal position, knees drawn up, thumbs tucked into clenched fists. But I don't uncurl.

DISCUSSION

In retrospect, was your decision to have no visitors the right one?
I think it was right for my family and friends.

How did lack of privacy in the radiotherapy room make you feel?
Vulnerable.

What needed to change?
Contact with a team would have provided improved opportunities for accessing information and support.

Explanations to patients convey respect, so can help them feel more in control and improve patient/professional relationships.[15]

Use of changing cubicles (or screens) and gowns (for example, specially designed gowns such as the 'Plymouth Gown' for radiotherapy to the breast) would help preserve patient dignity. A booklet written by lay members of the Clinical Oncology Patients' Liaison Group of the Royal College of Radiologists offers recommendations to enable medical staff to provide the best possible service.[16]

A patient-centred service would inform patients they could use two-way intercoms in radiotherapy rooms in an emergency.[17] International Atomic Energy Agency radiotherapy safety recommendations for 1998 (p.34) state: 'There should be audio communication from the patient during treatment.' www.inca.gov.br/pqrt/download/TECDOC_1040.pdf

---

Chapter 13

Birds of a feather
A bed by the window
That suits me fine!

Light seeps from the east
Before the paint's dry
Flooding wet into wet
And with every dawning
A gull comes battling across the sky

Blazing a trail
In the chill of morning:
The exhausting trip
(To the Corporation Tip?)
We both aim to survive
For just another day
But which will still be battling
When the other has flown away?

But for now, I'm so lucky
I've a wide screen view
Of my own 'Nature Watch'
And the changing hues of a canvas renewed
(On 'sky TV'!)

I've a bed by the window
And it means so much to me

All thought of sleep is abandoned. It doesn't matter. Why waste time sleeping when your shelf-life is limited?

Pale streaks appear in the dark sky, slanting in from the east, and for the first time I watch dawn break over this alien place. The process gathers pace, shades of grey giving way to ice green and grey tinged with pink, until suddenly it's full-blown morning and there's live action as a lone gull enters left, tipped one way and another by the wind. Determination keeps it on track. *Symbolic. I have the same resolve and intend to win my battle.*

Gradually, the ward comes to life and begins the routine of drug trolleys, food trolleys, nurses' flying spot checks and doctors' rounds. But the only person who actually comes to talk to me is a clerical officer with a list of questions. It's good to chat to her for a few minutes.

"Don't fight it, Mitzi," she advises, indicating the chemotherapy.

"Oh, I'm not. Don't worry, I welcome it." I wonder what it's like for her, working in this place of death.

Morning monotony is broken when a bundle of letters, get-well cards and presents arrive. Soon I'm surrounded by flowers, some in elaborate arrangements. Pretty soon my corner looks like a florist's shop. They are very beautiful, but I wish people would not spend so much money on me.

Later in the morning, a new patient is installed in the neighbouring bed and I smile briefly as I walk past on my way to the loo. My bum is getting very sore from diarrhoea and the internal pain at the tumour site is worsening, but there is no privacy for washing and I have to clean my bottom using toilet paper wetted with flushing water. Back on the ward, relatives sit ominously by the opposite bed. It's depressing. Too close to home.

Despite a reluctance to hear about my neighbour's illness, I can see she is anxious so I befriend her. Her name is Vera, she's in her seventies and worried in case her relatives won't visit because they would have to change buses three times. She hasn't any children and is pleased to share my family snaps.

She came in as an 'urgent admission', and hasn't brought any money, so I brighten her bedside with flowers and buy her a newspaper when the trolley arrives. This minor kindness prompts her to share a confidence: she has not had her bowels open for three weeks! *Does she mean three days?* My stomach lurches. Too much information! I'm wondering how to steer the conversation onto pleasanter matters when a nurse arrives to give her an enema.

They can't expect me to stay here while she performs! Stuff this communal living!

I grab lamppost and book and escape. The patients' sitting room is empty, and I've just settled down for a quiet read when two young men walk in, complete with lampposts, and turn on the TV. Both are bald. So young! Which cancer . . . what chance? Just as I realise I've read the same sentence three times, the foul stench of faeces hits my nostrils. I wonder if the air conditioning is bringing the smell from the toilets, or if one of the men has an overflowing colostomy bag. I can't offend them by walking out when they've just arrived, so pretend to blow my nose and surreptitiously breathe through a hankie.

"And now," announces the TV presenter, breaking through attempts to lose myself in the book, "it's time for 'Living With Dying'." A concerted groan goes up. One of the men switches channels, muttering, "Yes, we could really do with that."

It's an opportunity to leave. Outside in the corridor I fill my lungs and wonder where to go. Not back to the ward. Maybe I can find that glazed bridge I passed through with a nurse. Convinced I won't be missed for a while longer, I turn the corner and go exploring.

How good it feels to look down on greenery, flowers and birds. Pity there's nowhere to sit. I stand soaking up the real world as long as I can until nausea and weakness drive me back to the ward.

Vera's curtains are open. Her toileting has ceased. I smile briefly, but lie facing the window, breathing in the cold, fresh air to prevent having to listen to a description of the enema's effectiveness. Or otherwise.

At mealtimes, she has great difficulty feeding herself and constantly drops cutlery. The nurses are busy, so I retrieve things for her, but bending down increases my nausea. It's worse still when I try to eat. Hospital food tastes revolting. The nurse seems concerned that I'm not eating and I'm getting a little worried myself now.

"I came into hospital determined to fight cancer, but how can I fight, if I can't eat?" I ask in exasperation.

"Staff eat the same food as patients," she smiles, patiently.

How can they eat it? I need real, fresh food, not this reconstituted chemical catering concoction. She suggests I try some custard and the thought excites my taste buds – until the first spoonful. *It's custard . . . but not as you know it.* I don't think of blaming the chemotherapy.

The books I brought with me lie heaped upon the chair, unread. I write a few lines to friends and family, but can't concentrate. The ward fills with noisy visitors again. Feeling quite sick, I put my head under the covers to try to doze, but it's impossible. I try wandering up and down the corridor, but feel weak and ill and have to return to lie down.

Tea-time again. Relief as visitors thin out. No white bread again. I don't care. I'm so light-headed, I feel drugged. Oh, yes. I forgot. I am drugged. Ha! Ha! Drugged and dying. Or not. As the case may be. And time hanging. Such precious time, being frittered away in this dreadful place.

Nothing to do, but plenty of time to think – and it all crowds in on me.

Facing the Faceless
So will the emptiness envelop me
And with its cold embrace
Chase away the light?

Despair and loneliness encompass me
And, as I leave this race
Blot you from my sight?

I make the silent plea, "No tears for me"
And in this loveless place
I give up the fight?

Or will your hand be there, to comfort me
And give me strength to face
One last battle-site?

I'm alone in a cancer hospital, surrounded by dying patients in every ward, every floor, every wing of the building. More are admitted every day. The enormity of situation hits me. It's overwhelming. I'm facing death but no-one's talking about it. I have no concept of the timescale for treatment not working and imagine I might die in this first week. My death here would have as little significance as death in a remote land at the hands of the Chinese all those years ago. *If I die, will someone hold my hand, at last? Will I feel the solace of human touch?*

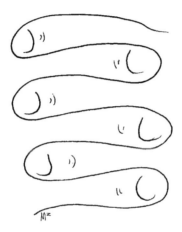

Figure 13.1 Solace.

Insight
So this is how the end will be
Lost and falling, endlessly
Crowding layers of ruthless dark
Obliterate

Or will my blindness help me see
Love's cold-store depository
Reveal friends' staunchness, as we part
Elucidate?

I'm lying here, trying to imagine what dying will be like. They don't tell you that. The taboo subject. I want to know what I might have to face. No more surprises! Being dead won't matter to me – because I'll be dead. The dying part might be more difficult. Will someone make sure I'm pain-free? I can't hear anyone screaming. That's hopeful.

What will my epitaph be? How about, 'She was very good at making bad decisions'? If only I can have one year. What haven't I done? Travel. Adventure. What else? Can't think . . . so tired . . . doesn't seem to matter that much any more. It's the ones left behind that suffer. Lucky to have been a mother of four. What difficulties might my children face? I am their champion, their protector. How can I cause them harm? The thought is unbearable.

Preconceptions, misconceptions
Pain and nausea, diarrhoea
Now I come to terms with dying
Conquering the final fear
But there's no-one here to listen
No-one who has learned to 'hear'

Even when they find me crying
(Picturing the ones left grieving
That's what needs the healing balm:
Mothers should protect their children
Buffer them, not cause them harm)
No-one uses the right questions

They see only fear of cancer
(I am made of sterner stuff!)
Even though they're really trying,
Kindliness is not enough

It's quiet now. People will hear if I cry. Feet into slippers, hoping the nurses won't notice my face as I pass, I make for the only spot hidden from their view – the chair behind the toilet door – but there's only a few moments of privacy.

"What are you crying about?" It's one of the nurses.

I've got cancer and I'm likely to die and what will my children do and how will they cope and how awful will it be for them . . . and . . . and . . . what the heck does she think I'm crying about!

"I don't know how I'll cope with being sick" I sniffle.

How odd! What I really want to talk about is my children.

"The type of drugs you are having don't always make people sick."

I'm malleable and need to believe her, but is this just a ploy, a psychological placebo to induce mind over matter?

Quite unwell this evening. Try watching television. Can't hear what's being said. Ears ringing with the din. Time for 'lights out' at last, or rather 'lights dimmed'. Curtains have masked the opposite bed all day. Emerging relatives look resigned. I try to convey sympathy when I catch their eye. Are they thinking that I could be next? Can't help wondering if there's a special ward for all terminally ill patients. And if this is it.

Charnel House?
Days and nights of unsought sharing
Rasping, gasping on display
Oxygen cylinders, rushing and clanking
Relatives' vigil: time to pray

Curtains closed for the conclusion
Starkly, in the new-born day
While the daily buzz continues
Stands the (briefly) empty bed
All around, the buzz continues
And nothing is said
Nothing is said

Minutes stretch into hours. Nurses patter, cylinders clank. Noises are magnified by the quiet of the night. There is greater urgency in the whispers. The coughing is relentless. I drop off eventually, the covers pulled over my head. And in the morning, wake to face an empty bed.

DISCUSSION

Why didn't you mention your eating and sleeping difficulties, or ask to talk to a dietician?
I didn't know I could ask to speak to a dietician. Anyway, I was going to be their best patient and couldn't be seen to be a wimp. I was in their hands.

So you expected to suffer?
Yes. Suffering had to be endured

What was it like to have no privacy for washing your bottom?
It was demoralising. Constant diarrhoea was already making me feel 'unclean', as well as sore.

Why do you think no-one talked about death and dying?
They were focussing on getting a positive outcome.

What effect did this have?
It created a surreal situation and barriers to communication.

What made you feel that dying in hospital would be comparable with dying in India?
Life seemed so cheap and death so familiar.

What needed to change?
Communication skills training would allow clinicians to discuss 'difficult' issues with patients.[18]
   Patients' dietary needs should be included as part of their care.[19]
   Patients need verbal and written information about ancillary services and other sources of help.

Chapter 14

Incongruity
Prisoner in an unbarred cell
Trapped by necessity
Yet, you smile and begin, "Well, isn't this nice!"
Disquiet, disparity
Words conflict with senses in this alien place
Overflowing with people
Wondering
All the poor people

"Swap you?" lies stillborn on my lips
Mocked by futility
Inanely, I grin
Words can't suffice
Shocked unreality
Look past the flowers to the stricken face
Among the poor people

Suffering
So many people

Impotent, sad, what help can I bring, freed from complacency?
Where to begin?
You pay the price
With pretence at normality
Self preservation, while running the race
For all the poor people
Lingering
Dying
Too many people

I try to concentrate on the changing sky, to find solace in its inconstant moods, a new painting dictated by time and weather. The gull passes on his morning trek. Maybe it's a different bird, but I pretend it's my special one.

The young doctor is a welcome diversion, but surprises me by exclaiming, "Ah! The first smile!"

I hadn't realised. "Sorry." *Why am I apologising again?*

He makes a note on his clipboard. So they note your first smile. Interesting! What else? I take note of them taking note.

The oncologist arrives later. He stands at the foot of the bed, all beaming smile and oozed confidence as I prepare for the 'How-are-you-fine' routine. He takes in the get-well cards and massed flowers with a sweeping glance that settles back on me.

"Well, isn't this nice!"

Swap you? I'm in this alien place, fighting death and I've just spent two days and nights listening to a dying patient trying to cough. *'Nice?'* It's mind-blowing.

I twitch a half-smile and try to see things from his viewpoint, but this continued lack of acknowledgement of my real situation is unnerving. It's all a game of pretence. *'Don't mention the war!'*

"How are you?"

"Fine." *There! Got that out of the way!*

He talks about the treatment. "And you've started radiotherapy?" He checks the clipboard.

"Mm . . ." *You know I have.*

"Might as well get them both started," he suggests with a broadening smile. To my super-charged antennae, the remark is thrown in unnecessarily, with affected nonchalance. It's the look the dog gives when it's just been sick on the sitting room carpet – that mixture of contrived innocence and apologetic guilt. He's trying to put me off the scent – of what?

He asks about my family and where my older children live. Perhaps he's concerned at my lack of visitors, or maybe he's just being sociable. At the mention of my husband, I can only mutter, "We are not close."

People change. Couples grow apart. Both must shoulder the blame, if blame there is. For some, ignoring a problem means it does not exist. Maybe this is one reason why the sense of unreality here hits me so starkly. I'm living a parallel charade.

"Any questions?"

Hoping to mirror his nonchalance, I manage, "Have I got it anywhere else?" My GP will have passed on my message about needing full information, so I'm expecting the truth.

"No."

It had been the merest hesitation, but it had stretched to infinity as he'd glanced away. Bells are tinkling again.

"You didn't look me in the eye when you said that."

There I go again. Blunt. Rude! Out of character – shocking myself! It takes enormous effort to be assertive, but my mouth takes over and says whatever is necessary to get at the truth. At least now he can't be in any doubt about my need for openness.

"Hrrrmph!" He swallows his amusement and relents. "All right then, we won't know until you've had a scan." *(Smile.)*

"When will that be?"

"Next Tuesday."

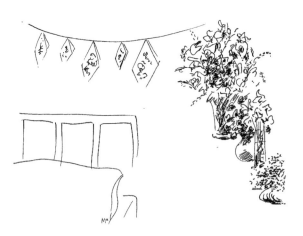

Figure 14.1 Incongruity.

56

Double disappointment slaps me down: he's still avoiding the truth – and there's almost a week to wait. I shouldn't have to prise out information. But I have to overlook this, try again to trust him. He is my lifeline, the only one with the expertise to save my life so, in one sense, his very presence is supportive, even though each encounter buffets me.

Sea of Tranquillity

There's no chance of a sleep
For the TVs all compete
Each channel with another
And the visitors' chatter
Competing with each other
Drowning out my lamp-post's
Inconsequential natter
With a deafening, battering
Shattering
Clatter
All the afternoon

So fingers in my ears
I dive for cover
As the volume's turned up
I attempt to smother
The din. But no-one
Can hear themselves speak
They're all shouting louder:
A din without a peak

More, much more than my pounding head can take
So it's 'walkies' for me
And my lamp-post on a lead
With pennies to squander
On postcards and pop
We go on an adventure
To the hospital shop

There's a queue, but no chair
And I can't stand in line
So I sit on the stair
And think, "They'd better be quick"
And then, "Where shall I be sick?"

My husband brings my dressing gown in the afternoon and there's a polite exchange of conversation. It's a difficult time for both of us. When he has gone, I feel very sick and lie down but, as usual, can't stand the noise, so ask to go to the hospital shop. Vera is distressed that she has no comb or mirror, so I aim to surprise her and also buy a birthday card for another patient. At the glass walk-way, I stop to watch the outside world, but nausea and weakness make me press on until I find the shop.

Vera is overjoyed with her presents and when the nurses give the 'birthday girl' my anonymous card it's a source of pleasure and curiosity for the rest of the afternoon.

After a fitful night, I wake to find a grey, blustery sky tossing the gull like a matchstick at sea. As the morning lengthens, the wind drops and the sky becomes leaden. Similarly featureless, the day stretches ahead, punctuated only by the ordeal of meal times, chemotherapy bag changes and trips to the loo. Sallying forth for radiotherapy becomes almost a highlight. I'm bored, yet don't feel well enough to do anything. This is what it must be like in an old people's home.

Pressure Point
Well out of sight, all curtained and contained,
The heartaches never known to me, the horrors never dreamed,
For you, are just mundane
You live the other side of life's uneven game

And when the day is done
Is there someone who can read
The numbness seeping through
Someone who lets you offload, to keep you whole?
For how can anyone be drenched in death
And not implode?

So have you built a wall of glass, so thick
That tragedy can't penetrate or break and nothing sticks or marks
And you don't care?

Or are your open sores well dressed, the abscess, undisplayed
And is the sorrow locked below
The plate-glass window
'Just for show'?

Laughter peals out from the nurses' station. I don't begrudge them sharing a joke. They are kindness itself and, working in this place, they deserve some amusement. I wonder how they cope with all the tragedy and trauma. Yet it's unsettling; another incongruity. Even their background chatter is difficult to listen to: their normality, in my world of abnormality. It's because there's no acknowledgment of the seriousness of my situation, *our* situation – the plight of all these people. No-one comes to talk to me. *Is cancer spreading throughout my body? I wish the scan could be done now.*

I'm so lonely, I'm even envious of patients having their temperatures taken! The monotony is relieved when I see an air bubble in my chemotherapy line and get the chance to press my nurse-call bell. Such excitement! *You die if an air bubble enters your bloodstream, don't you? Will I die before they get to me?* They smile tolerantly at my ignorance. There's a special safety valve. Back to boredom.

At lunch-time, they offer build-up drinks, but the thought of milk induces nausea. Never mind, I could do with losing some weight. I manage a little yoghurt, then stand looking out at the world through the glass-panelled door at the far end of the ward. On the way back to bed, a lovely young woman in her late thirties starts chatting. She tells me she has breast cancer, but her skin is not healing properly. "Not a good sign," she says, adding mysteriously that, as a nurse, she knows too much. *What does it mean? What does she know? How much is 'too much'?* I don't like to press her, to intrude, but I'm surprised to learn her daughter spends every day here with her. *Is it because she is dying?* When I mention my sleeping problem, she asks if I have a relaxation and visualisation tape, but when she realises I don't know what she is talking about, her daughter promises to copy one for me. Apparently, there are walkman headsets on this ward (but locked away in a cupboard). Elsewhere there is a library and group relaxation classes are held regularly. Nobody has mentioned any of this.

Meeting her sets me thinking. I look through my photographs for comfort. Should I have asked my children to visit, or even to stay all day? I don't want them to miss classes, but if the treatment doesn't work these could be my last few days – and I will have lost my last chance to be with them.

I'm very lucky to have such supportive children and friends. Flowers, cards and letters keep arriving. I share them with Vera. My corner becomes ever more floral; the oncologist's beam stretches wall to wall.

By day, the chemotherapy pump is my friend, its magic potion waging war on my cancer. But in the quiet of the night, its rhythmical ticks count off the minutes. Ticking my life away. And almost every waking second, I think about the scan. *Has it spread to my brain? Will I go mad? Will I go mad, waiting to know if I'm going to go mad . . .?*

DISCUSSION

What could be more normal than remarking, 'Well, isn't this nice?'
It would have been entirely normal – if the situation had been normal.

You felt information was being withheld?
Yes. After so much misinformation, I was extra sensitive to their body-language.

What effect did this have on you?
Lack of trust fuelled uncertainty and stress.

Why didn't you challenge them?
I felt intimidated, disempowered by illness and my 'patient' role.

You felt you had to go along with them?
Yes. I became drawn into their game of pretence.

Why do you keep mentioning their smiles?
The insincerity was hard to take. Later, when I came across a doctor's admission that they (the profession) 'adopt an artificially cheerful exterior signalling 'don't ask serious questions',[20] it was immensely important to me.

Would you have preferred them to look serious?
I appreciated supportive smiles, but not those designed to cover deceit.

What was the effect of the false cheerfulness?
It blocked serious discussion.

What needed to change?
Patients need:
» instant truth, not tailored, protective responses
» a clear understanding of what they are facing
» to have the seriousness of their situation acknowledged
» to be respected

Chapter 15

Yesterday stretched endlessly, like the ninth month of pregnancy. But Saturday is here at last, I've had a blood test and the results were fine, so I'm going home! Or at least, I am once this chemo bag has emptied. My eldest son's coming to fetch me.

I scribble 'woz yur' beneath my name card at the head of the bed, then wonder why I did that. A gentle protest against institutional anonymity? A need to leave my mark? I have survived the first week, but when the sheets are changed and all traces of me are removed, it will be as if I have never existed. As if I had died.

Willing the chemo level to drop has little effect. As I reflect on the past week, I realise powerful images have already reduced former memories to fast-fading watercolours.

I've never managed to speak to a young Asian woman across the aisle. Coping with my own symptoms and those of my immediate neighbours has been enough. How pathetic! Perhaps she can't speak English. Imagine having cancer and not understanding what is said to you. (Years later, I still recall her stricken face.)

Despite everything negative about being in hospital, I suppose I have formed an attachment for this place where they have been saving my life. I feel such empathy for the doctors, nurses and radiotherapists and great admiration that they have the resilience to deal with death and dying on a daily basis, yet have shown me nothing but patience and kindness. Although home is where I long to be, I know things could get much tougher. I'll be fighting it alone, within the stress of a broken relationship.

My thoughts break off as a figure strides into the ward and fills it with his presence. My son's careful hug and kiss send comfort crashing through my body. Even though the chemo bag's not quite empty, the nurse removes the cannula and says I can leave.

I feel like tissue paper. Dressing is frustratingly slow. I surround Vera with most of my flowers and give her a last, poignant kiss. She's going to a hospice. She thinks it's for 3 weeks.

"We hope we won't see you again!" smile the nurses as I bid them a brief 'goodbye', trying not to show how much I want to get away. How can I thank them adequately? I want to hug them, but they might not like it.

Crossing the hospital threshold is like escaping from the constraints of a disempowering dream-world. The lazy March sun caresses my upturned face for a moment, but it's no match for the Arctic wind streaking through my clothes and lashing tears from my eyes. Soon, I'm tucked into my son's car and leaving the hospital far behind. Although elated, I'm grappling with guilt and concern for patients who may never go home and staff who will be there tomorrow and every day.

I feel at least ninety and am strangely super-sensitive. I suppose it's the effect of the chemotherapy but, as rough road surfaces increase the vehicle's vibrations, it feels as if each individual cell in my body is being irritated. My son ignores irate drivers and slows to a snail's pace. The protracted journey takes almost 2 hours.

Home at last – to a welcome of wagging tails and doggy grins as I half fall out of the car. It's so good to hug my children. But indoors, I'm soon shivering. The inadequate central heating isn't even turned on and in my weakened state I'm feeling the cold far more than usual. A friend, Frances, has laid a fire in the grate, but it's slow to give out any heat. Shivering violently, I fill a hot-water bottle and collapse onto a chair.

The utility room, in the old stable block adjacent to the kitchen, has been my bedroom for several months. There is no ceiling and at night I have been able to see stars through a tear in the roofing felt. The oil-fired boiler gives off more fumes than heat, the brick walls are not plastered and there's no damp proof course, but here, away from the main part of the house, I have found some sort of peace. Now my priority will have to be warmth.

Perceptively, Frances suggests using the sitting room as my bedroom and helps set the bed against the radiator, opposite the window. I shall watch village life across the green, like a vicarious pensioner. The downstairs loo a few steps away becomes my private en suite and the dining room, a sitting room.

Gita, my next-door neighbour, pops round and announces she's taken part of her annual leave for the express purpose of driving me to radiotherapy next week. "Can't let you go there on your own," she says, emphatically. It would be churlish to refuse her sacrifice, but I've been so looking forward to the independence of driving myself. We compromise: I'll drive and she will accompany me.

'Never stand when you can sit. Never sit when you can lie . . .' my grandmother's words echo in my head. So of course I won't sit until I am about to fall down. Later, I even try to take the dogs for a walk, just to show how strong I am.

As we pass through the orchard, the cat leaps out, pats one of the dogs on the nose in passing and continues vertically up an apple tree. The dogs turn away in embarrassment and go haring down the field. The horse snorts in surprise, then joins the chase, the pony hot on its heels. I feel too weak to deal with their boisterous antics so walk safely in parallel through the vegetable garden, deafened by the insistent cries of hungry nestlings and intoxicated by the scents of wild flowers and crushed grass. It's a world away from sterile hospital air – and cancer. Even the muck heap smells sweet! I'd intended to climb the gate and wander down the green lane, but I've ground to a halt. Never mind. It's been sheer heaven.

That night as I lie awake, consultations replay in my head in endless circles. Hesitations, evasions, lies, accumulated 'things that do not fit' nag at me for explanation. I practise relaxation techniques with my tape and finally fall asleep. It does not seem to matter that I'm wide awake 4 hours later.

Chapter 16

The weekend is over too soon and the daily hospital trek begins, but there's only one more day to wait for the scan. Today I'll see the consultant as well as have radiotherapy, while my neighbour visits a friend on a ward. Although the clinic waiting area is full, it's not long before I'm ushered into the consulting room. Perhaps they know I have a long drive home. The beaming smile accompanies our 'How-are-you-fine' preamble.

"Any problems?" he asks.

I shake my head. *No problems. I'm coping you see. I'm strong. You can give me all the information there is to give.*

He repeats what he's already told me about the treatment. There will be three more weeks' radiotherapy, a two week break before two more weeks' radiotherapy to the groin area, followed by another two-week break. Then the radioactive implants: six wires threaded needle-like through the tumour under general anaesthetic and connected to a radioactive source for sixty hours, which will necessitate another short stay in hospital.

The implants sound scary, but I'm reasonably confident because I won't be awake when they are inserted. The greatest challenge might be in having to lie very still for so long. I'm looking forward to the two week break, though. Something to aim for. Perhaps I can go away.

"And you've got your appointment for the CT scan, tomorrow?" he checks.

Oh yes! I nod – and doubt I'll sleep at all tonight.

"Any questions?"

I'm full of them. Mostly stupid. How do I know what to ask when I know absolutely nothing about cancer or treatments? It's like trying to understand quantum physics, without even a science O'-level. But I hope the constant questioning will make him realise I'm capable of dealing with scary information.

"Is this one of a series of treatments?" *Credit me. I really want to understand.*

Cancer patients have second and third courses of chemotherapy. Are they going to spring more treatments on me?

"No. This is your lot!" he asserts, still beaming.

So I only get one chance. Why can't I have more treatment if necessary – because it costs too much? Because I'm too old?

"So what happens – if it doesn't work? Do you start – chopping me up?"

Breathless sentences – also delivered with a smile. *See! I can talk about these things* . . . But he's not smiling now.

"We'll see how it goes."

That was unfair of me. He can't be flippant, so I shouldn't be. But I want to know. Judging from his reaction, I seem to have touched a nerve. Mm . . . must watch my step in future.

A nurse escorts me to the radiotherapy waiting area. I don't have long to wait. The production line is in full swing. Radiotherapy staff are always kind and chatty. They introduce themselves along with any students and explain precisely what is going to happen before they do anything. As they check that radiotherapy guidance ink marks on my skin are still visible, they ask what I've been doing over the weekend and express a keen interest in my hobby, watercolour painting. One says she would like to take it up herself and asks me to bring in some of my work to show them. It's incredible that they can deal with an endless stream of people, yet always manage to take a personal interest in me.

Treatment doesn't take long, but it seems an age when you're trying to keep still, hold your breath and hold onto your dignity. Afterwards, I set off to find my neighbour and take the stairs rather than the lift to prove to myself (and anyone around) that I can still do it. When I drop by my old ward to thank the person who gave me the relaxation tape, there's someone else in 'my' bed and Vera has gone. I can't bear to look.

Exhaustion swamps me as we walk back to the car park. I need to lie down, but there's a forty-five mile drive ahead. It's good to have company. When we get back I have to lie down. Diarrhoea has been worsening each day and my insides feel raw most of the time. Even passing wind is very painful. Going to the loo (passing a motion) is now excruciating. Although there is little solid matter, it's like having vinegar poured onto a wound that's being stretched in two directions. The pain stays with me long after I've finished. Co-proxamol has little effect and also makes my head spin. Because I need to be able to drive I take it only in the evening and at night.

Tension at home is unbearable, so I take the dogs for a potter around the top field. Bedtime allows me to drop the pretence of being 'fine'. Practising with the relaxation tape usually helps me take some control, countering the dragging ache inside my body and the bombardment in my brain, until I tip into a short sleep. But not tonight. Thoughts of what the CT scan might reveal, fill my head. The grandfather clock strikes 3.00 am, but I must have dropped off, for the next thing I know it's time to get dressed. Scan day has arrived.

DISCUSSION

Why were you flippant?
I was trying to raise the possibility of treatment failure in a light-hearted way.

His reaction surprised you?
Yes. It seemed failure was not an option. If we did not talk about it, it would not happen – just like personal issues at home.

Treatment failure was seen as personal failure?
That was my impression.

Did anyone ask you if Co-proxamol was effective?
No. The consultant always asked if I had any problems, but I felt I had to be seen to be coping in order to get information.

Were you told that pain relief medication was most effective when taken regularly?
No. And I didn't realise my body would probably adjust to the side effects.

Were you told it might help counter diarrhoea?
No. The side effects of medication were not discussed.

What needed to change?
Patients need good quality information in order to be in control of their situation.

Open sharing of information improves the consultation.[21]

Patient concordance is likely to improve when patients are given sufficient understandable information.[15]

Clinicians need to talk about pain and ask specific questions.

Chapter 17

Half truth is no truth
Fencing the questions week after week
She's only a patient
Unable to cope with the extent of the mess
Mustn't let her calculate, evaluate
She mustn't guess
She mustn't see the whole picture

Let her think we rate her chances high
That she, probably, won't die
Paint in bright colours the dullest of scenes
Paint it by numbers, puzzle and scheme
Oblivious to the silent screams of mounting frustration

Bending the truth 'for the patients' sake'
Tell only as much as you think she can take

My heightened awareness helps me see
But you blunt the edge of reality
I'll savour my time
But to what degree
If I can't taste the finality?

This isn't how it has to be: by holding back you impoverish me
No matter how dreadful, no matter how sad
No matter how great the Medical Might
I should have the sole copyright.
I need to have the whole picture

The drive this morning was tiring and stressful. The impending CT scan encouraged speed, while blinding spray from swaying caravans and countless kamikazi lorries on the dual carriage-way counselled patience.

Now I'm lying here, about to pass through a ring of metal that will take numerous images of my body. Shallow breathing is helpful for once as I try to keep absolutely still. I know it won't hurt and I can't wait to know the truth, but I'm still nervous. Silly, isn't it?

I can see them through a glass panel as they operate the machine, the young doctor and someone else. I return his smile. *What are you seeing? Has it spread to my brain? Am I riddled with it?*

When it's over I ask, quickly, "Has it spread anywhere else?" But I'm disappointed.

"You'll get the results in clinic," he says.

Clinic! That's not until Friday – another three days – and nights. But they know now! Other people have more information about my body than I do. Don't they realise it's the uncertainty that's unbearable? No matter how bad things are, I need to know my real situation and be able to come to terms with it. My body, my cancer, but I can't see the pictures. I'm only a patient.

During the week I bring in a couple of paintings to show the radiotherapy 'girls', but they're very busy and only glance cursorily at them. I realise their earlier enthusiasm had been encouragement, not genuine interest and sink into my shell.

By the time Friday arrives, the car seems to know its own way to the hospital. Apart from increasing pain, this week has been quite manageable. Soon, I'm sitting half naked on the examination couch, covered by a small sheet. Now, at last, I'll learn the scan results. Accompanying the oncologist is a nurse and also another young doctor I haven't seen before, whose permanent lighthouse beam smile puts others' in the shade. I'm expecting to hear the results straight away, but the consultation follows the set routine. *Why aren't they telling me? It must be really bad news.*

"How are you?"

"Fine."

How can he bear the boredom of asking the same thing time after time? We progress through the familiar questions about bowel movements and such-like, but nobody asks about the pain. I expected the treatment to be hard, but didn't know it would include this level of increasing pain. He must know what the treatment does to people, so I can't complain, or be seen to be weak, or he'll think I'm not coping and give me even less information. He examines my stomach, lower abdomen and groin areas – looking for more lumps I guess. My stomach is as hard as iron. It seems to amuse him.

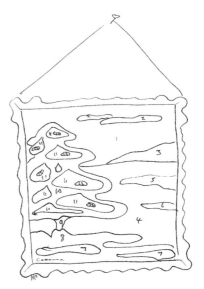

Figure 17.1 Whole picture.

"Just relax," he says, smiling. Small chance! It's bad enough just being here. Being looked at in such a penetrating fashion reduces me to 'specimen'. And today, any minute, I'm going to learn the scan results. I'm totally rigid with anticipation.

Finally, he says, "Right, turn over and we'll just take a look."

I'm getting used to having my bare butt examined, and one buttock raised to check how my skin is standing up to the radiotherapy. It's doing wonders for my inhibitions.

But the heart-crushing wait to hear the worst must be pushing my blood-pressure through the roof.

"Any questions?" he asks, sitting there, beaming at me.

I can't believe it! The consultation is ending and they're not even going to mention the scan results! Am I supposed to have forgotten about it? Do they think I don't want to know?

I'm locked in eye contact, immobilised by incredulity and 'need to know'.

"Scan?" – spat out, breathlessly – is all I can manage. From the corner of my eye, I note the nurse's flicker of alarm. Stress is off the scale. The very air is crackling. *Perhaps he sees my incoherence as 'fear of cancer'.* There's an elastic pause.

"There are two *small* ones, behind the main one" he concedes, in carefully measured tones, *(accent on 'small', the smile overstretched, unconvincing)* rounding off quickly with, ". . . but we expected that." *Oh! That's all right then!*

I need to see for myself, but asking will suggest mistrust. There's no spare breath for talking.

"C'n-I-see?"

As he flicks slowly through the scan pictures, I sit frozen, staring hypnotically. There lie the answers I need. I note how carefully he picks one – *the least frightening?*

What he hands me shows three white blobs in an oval slice. He identifies the middle one as my bottom. I can't see any 'small ones behind the main one' and guess they are the other two blobs on each side.

"Which is left . . . which right?" I need my glasses, but I can't take up his time to get them. He indicates 'R' and 'L' on the film, but doesn't explain anything. It's like drawing hen's teeth.

I want to know all about it. *Why don't they just offer me all the images? Why is it so hard to find out anything? Don't they realise how stressful this is?* But I'm shrinking.

Silence. They all stare, waiting for me to finish. Time's up. There's a waiting room full of patients beyond the door. I need to know precisely where I have cancer, to be able to understand my situation and fight it. But asking to see more slides will show doubt – tantamount to calling him a liar. I just can't do it and hand back the picture, little realising I will regret this for years to come.

When we reach the car, I draw the scan picture from memory. I need something solid, some reference point to help to put this thing in its place. Now at least I know it's on both sides of my pelvis. On the way home, Gita agrees it was a peculiar comment and seems distressed about the extra tumours, while I'm more concerned about what I haven't seen.

DISCUSSION

Why did you think you would have the scan results straight away?
A doctor was watching the scan pictures being taken. I thought he could tell me what he saw.

Why do you think they did not offer you all the pictures?
They thought they were protecting me.

How did that make you feel?
Stressed, frustrated and controlled.

How did 'but we expected that' make you feel?
I felt like exploding! It was a substitute for an explanation, like dismissing a child with 'because I say so'. Obfuscation seemed to be second nature to them, yet they were expecting blind trust.

How did you feel when you realised you would not be able to see all the scan pictures?
There was a great sense of loss. I had been so close to the tangible proof I needed.

You were frightened cancer might have spread?
Obviously that thought was frightening, but my need for truth was paramount and they seemed so reluctant to tell me anything. It felt like a nightmare cat and mouse game that I could never win.

Never win?
I could never get them to realise I could deal with full information.

How did you feel when you learned cancer had spread to both sides of your pelvis?
It was an incredible relief to gain even this much reliable knowledge. It is difficult to explain the depth of my 'need to know'. I was in an information desert. Anything was better than uncertainty.

What needed to change?
A booklet written by lay members of the Clinical Radiology Patients' Liaison Group of the Royal College of Radiologists (a companion to that mentioned earlier on good practice in radiotherapy departments) offers recommendations to enable medical staff to provide the best possible service.[22]
  Patients need:
» to be warned in advance when to expect diagnostic results
» to be enabled to discuss the implications
» to be offered results as a right not a privilege
» to be offered copies of results to take away
» to be heard.

Chapter 18

Nothing to rely on
Consultations
Constant replay
Every flicker of the eyes
Discrepancies, anomalies
Every nuance, hesitation

Consultations and lack of information cause more anxiety than the cancer. They replay over and over in my head, every point teased out and chewed over until the next meeting. I have started making notes of everything that has happened and write down the conversations after each consultation, trying to discover why information is being withheld and whether my suspicions are imaginary. That night, sleep is a nightmare of fractured dreams. But insomnia doesn't matter. When I'm awake, I know I'm alive.

The hospital trek has become something to look forward to, an outing. It's good to be out of the house, even though the journey is painful and I swap one stress for another. Skirting towns and cities, the ring road passes through rolling hills, lifting my spirits. The prospect of death has given me an enhanced appreciation of nature's beauty. Simple things confer disproportionate pleasure: rooks gathering twigs; a scattering of spring flowers; horses bucking as they shake off the frosty night. These things will still be here next spring, renewing their dance to the earth's rhythm – with or without me.

Although exhausted after treatment, I avoid going straight home. Most friends are at work, but some are sick or retired and for them, I discover, my very presence now has healing powers! I'm a good listener and people pour out their troubles, but inevitably finish by saying, '. . . but my problems are nothing compared with yours . . .' My closeness to death puts their situation into perspective and they seem much happier. I enjoy black humour.

But I don't know how much longer I can cope with this pain. When I first went to my GP with symptoms, it was because I felt the pain was unbearable, but it has increased greatly since then. The dull ache in my groin and left side is now strong enough to keep me awake at night, although it's nothing like the agony of defecation. When I lie on my right side, gravity pulls at my intestines, which feel as though they are suspended from an area of rawness. I change position often.

It's hurtful that few friends call. Perhaps they find cancer too difficult to deal with and don't know what to say. I wandered across the village green yesterday and saw one of my neighbours from a distance. When she noticed me, she tucked her head down and hurried away. I understand, but feel an outcast. I have learned to value friends. Those up to the challenge mean more to me than they could realise.

On Saturday, my daughter drives me to town, hoping to help me find some information about anal cancer. But by the time I've walked from the car park to the bookshop, I feel too sick and weak to stand. Shops don't have chairs these days. The old and sick are not a commercial proposition – no-one caters for their needs any more. There's a queue at the counter so, ignoring the stares of curious onlookers, I collapse onto the stairs and try to scan the bookshelves from there. There are books on bowel cancer, but nothing on anal cancer. When the queue drifts away, an enquiry at the counter is equally unsuccessful, but the mention of anal cancer seems to prematurely empty the shop. For a mad moment I contemplate walking up the high street shouting, 'Anal cancer! Anal cancer!' Ah! The power of the (possibly) terminally ill . . .

DISCUSSION

What needed to change?
One size does not fit all. Patients with rarer cancers need information, as well as those with common cancers.

Patients who want information should be offered specific details about their cancer, and sign-posted to further sources. Providing written information to patients can save time for healthcare providers. Website printouts are economical, but may need researching. Skinner and Springham, writing in *Quality in Primary Care*,[23] describe web-based tools that enable users to judge the reliability of sites and give a few examples of the many patient-friendly information websites available, such as www.labtestsonline,[24] a peer-reviewed resource that explains diagnostic tests in lay terms.

Chapter 19

It's week 3. I'm not so cocky now. Going to the toilet is real agony half a dozen times a day or more. I pass little except blood and slime, but the tumour site feels raw, passing even the smallest amount of faeces burns, while violent spasm and wind stretch my insides. I flush the loo to mask my groans.

It takes me about an hour and a half to have a bath and get dressed every day, so it's a good job the radiotherapy appointments are always late morning. I just can't hurry. The car journey is getting increasingly painful too. The soft seat hurts more than a wooden chair. There is never any room to park near the hospital entrance and it's getting more and more difficult to walk up the slope from the lower car park. I don't know why, but I'm puffing like an old man and have to stop several times to get my breath.

In the mornings, I have a little appetite and feel least nauseous, but I dare not eat anything in case I fill my pants in the car or the waiting room, so I take a couple of cream crackers to nibble on the way home, but feel too tired and sick to eat much more for the rest of the day. Defecation has become increasingly unpredictable and the possibility of a traffic jam is never far from my thoughts. I can no longer tell the difference between needing to pass wind and needing to defecate. The spectre of my bum oozing faeces just before treatment, or while being examined, haunts and demoralises me. Day after day, I wash my bottom in the hospital toilet, then sit in the crowded waiting area in an agony of apprehension, hoping one of the two toilets will be vacant if I need it. *What if faeces leaks down my legs as I stand . . . I am an Untouchable. Should I be ringing a bell? 'Unclean! Unclean!'*

The treatment is not supposed to hurt, but as I lie here shivering, the pain in my insides is affected by the cold. Each time they insert the metal sheet beneath me for the second treatment I have the sensation of an internal ice burn – as if an ice-lolly has ripped off a layer of skin. Staff look uncomfortable when I mention this. They have a job to do and I guess it's unfair of me to talk about what effect their treatment is having, but I realise I'll have to ask them to get me some better pain relief soon. However, it's not until after radiotherapy on Tuesday that I'm able to pluck up courage to mention it. Although we've formed a good relationship, it's so hard to ask them. I'm a failure.

"How does it feel?" they ask.

"Like there's a teazle stuck up my bottom," I tell them. "When I go to the loo it's like passing shards of glass." I'm not exaggerating. They look distressed and say they'll 'see what they can do'.

I'm in agony on the toilet that evening but next day nobody mentions my request. *Surely they can't have forgotten!* But I can't broach the subject. This is the forbidden area. *'Don't mention the war!'* repeats in my head. I drive home with tears pouring down my face.

There is a continual grinding pain in the whole of my lower abdomen. When I defecate, the pain defies description. I squash a toilet roll and thrust it into my mouth to mask the groans and to give me something to bite down on. No matter what they think of me, I will have to ask them again tomorrow. I feel so ashamed, but I just can't stand any more of this. The pain is frightening.

Forcing myself to confront them, I ask shamefacedly, "Please, did you ask about getting some pain relief?" *I must not leave this hospital without something to relieve the agony.* They look at each other. Then they look at the floor.

"We're very sorry," they say. "He said there's nothing else you can have."

The homeward journey is blinded by tears. On the loo that night, pain reaches new heights. Biting on a toilet roll is not enough. Ridiculous in my efforts to cope, I begin banging my head on the wall.

DISCUSSION

There were only two toilets in the waiting area?
Yes. Concerned nurses circulated a short survey, asking for patients' comments. I wrote 'they are very clean', when what I wanted to say was 'radiotherapy can cause diarrhoea – people are suffering because there are not enough toilets'.

What stopped you?
I felt so indebted to staff, I could not make any sort of criticism.

Did anyone offer you incontinence pads?
No. No-one enquired about my faecal difficulties and it was not a subject I could raise.

Why didn't you ask the oncologist for better pain relief?
I had to put on a front – show him I could cope in order to get honest information.

But other staff would tell him you couldn't cope with the pain.
Maybe I thought others could get the message across that I was strong and coping. It was too hard to admit my failure to him face to face. I was not thinking logically. Perhaps starvation and pain warp the mind?

You really banged your head on the wall?
Yes. The pain was too terrible to do nothing.

What needed to change?
I needed
» an advocate – a specialist nurse – to ensure my needs were met
» effective pain relief[25]
» dedicated patient parking close to the hospital entrance
» adequate numbers of clean, regularly-serviced toilets in the Out-Patient Department

Chapter 20 ━━━

Transmogrify
No more feigned interest in my yesterdays, no more pretence
You cannot share
The precious moments that are mine
No more small-talk about the weekend jaunts
You cannot care
Too many passing through

My body you may jellify
I acquiesce, I understand the need
But please, no more attempts to jollify
Today, just let me be
So skip the inane pleasantries
The 'hairdresser's chit chat'
Emulsify me if you must
But leave my thoughts to me

(And know immediate regret
Mindful of the task that's set
Harsh words I cannot justify
So wretchedly, with deep remorse
I vainly try
To mollify)

During the Friday clinic, the oncologist measures the lump in my groin with a pair of callipers.

"It's going already," I offer brightly.

"Have you been feeling it?" he asks. "You shouldn't feel it."

I check the fixed smile, uncertainly. Had I imagined that avuncular 'don't worry your little head about it' edge to the tone? I may be childlike in my need for total honesty; in my dependence, obstinacy, pride and need for their approval – but not in blind acceptance. *My lump, my body, my death. I'll feel it when I want to!*

The rest of the clinic follows the set routine, done in precisely the same order with precisely the same words, 'How are you . . .?

Any problems . . .? and 'Right, turn over, and we'll just take a look' and 'Any questions?'. How boring for him. I'm in despair, but can't raise the issue of pain relief. I tell myself they would relieve my pain if they could. There can't be any suitable short term pain relief that would help, yet allow me to stay conscious during defecation and be capable of driving. And if a specialist can't suggest anything, it's no good asking my GP. I'm on my own.

The weekend is a swill of pain and replayed consultations. Monday sees me back on the treadmill for my fourth week of treatment. Life has become an increasingly difficult endurance test, the journey to hospital, something to dread. At every bump in the road, pain spears through me. As fatigue engulfs me, I drive faster – eighty, ninety – hoping I won't kill anyone, but desperate to get there.

By the time I reach home after treatment I'm totally drained and need to lie down, but feebly exercise my legs to maintain muscle tone. 'Walking the dogs' has reduced to a slow plod down the lane. If I can put one foot in front of another, I can walk. It helps reduce the discomfort of bloat. Trudge, trudge, plod, plod, '*A Mitzi-Bird does not give up . . . a Mitzi-Bird does not give up . . .*' Once the children get back from school I try to assume a healthy 'front'. We don't talk about what might happen. We are protecting each other with a wall of silence, just like at the hospital.

My daughter cooks the evening meal, but I can't eat and I'm too tired for it to matter. Sometimes I can eat a whole yoghurt if I take it slowly, but usually I manage half. It should be enough to keep me alive. Anyway, more food would mean more poo and more pain.

"Perhaps I'd be better off eating only soup," I suggest to a nurse, one day, hoping for advice. "You'll be in trouble if you do," she replies, darkly and I wonder if my intestines would stick together.

Each day I think the pain of defecation can't get any worse, but each day it hits a new high. My insides still feel raw half an hour later. I've had four children, my first born in India without any type of analgesia, even for episiotomy. I thought I knew what pain was. Now I know what real agony is. Even the pre-defecation signal is a searing pain. Toilet paper dampened with anaesthetizing cold water is all I can bear to dab on my outer skin, and it comes away covered in pinpricks of blood. Whatever the radiotherapy does to kill cancer, it doesn't magic it away. My GP sends some anaesthetic gel but the tiniest amount burns the exterior anal skin. I can't possibly use it inside me. There is nothing to relieve my pain.

Radiotherapy staff are just as meticulous and kind as before, but I feel too tired to play along. They talk to me as if they care, but now it feels as though they don't. There's a gulf between us. It must be

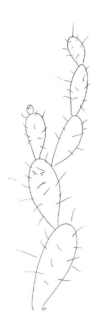

Figure 20.1 Prickly pear.

my fault they don't take me seriously, because I can't communicate effectively. Conflict builds as the week progresses. When they ask what I've been doing, I can only manage, "Not-a-lot." Words are too heavy and breath too scarce for chat.

They leave me alone after that. Leave me to batter myself with remorse at my brusqueness. They've been particularly kind, but I can't bear the insincerity of this place. Wanting to make amends, I call into a roadside supermarket on the way home and next day present them with a cactus plant and an apology for being so prickly.

Everything is done in slow motion. I'm drunk with light-headedness and frustratingly weak. My hip joints hurt as I haul myself upstairs for the morning bath, which now takes twice as long as normal.

The sitting room is a tip. Cards, letters and dying flowers fill the mantelpiece, donated magazines litter the floor. Four walls have become a prison and even the most delightful view can pall. As I've become more housebound, I've realised how important it is to have something to look forward to – a friend to call, a favourite TV programme, anything to combat the bleakness of empty days and enforced immobility. Despite heavy family commitments and full time work, Frances comes to clean the house whenever she can.

Kath often calls and fills the evening with amusing stories about the surgery and village life.

I still can't eat. I still can't sleep. I try to paint some wilted flowers, but the effort is too much. The thought of staying with old friends in Wiltshire during my two-week break sustains me.

DISCUSSION

Why did you think their lack of openness might be your fault?
My vocabulary had shrunk. I was breathless, incoherent and inarticulate. I could not blame them for assuming my stress was due to fear of cancer and trying to protect me.

What needed to change?
Patients need to be enabled to talk about their pain.
   Pain should be acknowledged and effective palliation offered.[26]

Chapter 21

Open book
Questions answered with a question
Gather thoughts and buy some time
For invention
"Black is white"
(You must believe me)
Underlining, with a smile

Something I forgot to mention –
Want to know how I divine your intention?
Want to know the telltale signs?

Momentarily, you 'lose it'
Fleetingly, you look aside
Just before the 'reassurance'
When you dare to meet my eyes

As the end of the four week treatment approaches, I decide to check that my planned holiday will not cause inconvenience.

"Is it all right with you if I go away?"

The oncologist looks aside before rearranging his smile and asking, "Where to?"

Why does it matter where I go? But the eyes had said it all. And once again the nurse had flashed a look of alarm, before studying the floor.

"I haven't decided," I return, suspecting they have no interest in 'where', and spontaneously deciding to play them at their game.

"I'm afraid you're going to be a bit ill," he admits, somewhat reluctantly. "It will be rather like 'flu'."

A 'bit' ill? Single syllables for the village idiot? They've known about this all along, but kept it from me. Would they have mentioned it at all, if I hadn't asked? Trust becomes increasingly elusive. In their game, with its ever-changing rules, I've slid down the snake and have to start climbing ladders all over again.

"Any questions?"

Yes, oh, yes! Why didn't you tell me this, weeks ago? Why didn't you warn me about the pain? Can't you acknowledge that treatments cause harm? Who are you really trying to protect – me or yourself? And what else haven't you told me?

More stillborn questions. Help! I'm locked in a game where meeting their expectations means being unable to express my needs. Questions are a wasted exercise. Despondently, I crumple the list in my hand

---

DISCUSSION

How did you feel when you learned you were going to be ill?
The prospect didn't upset me. Losing my holiday was disappointing. But far worse was my disappointment in them, for not sharing this earlier. No-one seemed to understand what this 'protection' was doing to me.

What needed to change?
There needed to be an end to paternalism.[27]

Chapter 22 ▬

Next!
Insect, trapped, exposed and bare
Tipped from a jar to be studied there

Specimen
Alone, defenceless, hemmed in tight
Pit yourself against the might of Medical Right

Crowding of people
Lock the cell door
Prepare for the onslaught

Barrage of questions
Probing of hands
Scrutinize, dehumanise
Laser-beam eyes make a meal
But no one asks, "How does it feel?"

Grinning faces, floating, gloating
While pain sears
I can't speak
But I won't give them the tears

(Poetic licence: I could not prevent tears pouring down my cheeks, but I would not sob.)

The Friday clinic in the fourth week of treatment begins in the same order and with precisely the same words as the now familiar routine. The consultant hoists up his 'trust in me' beam and it's smiles all round from the young clinic doctor and nurse. They are a kind, caring bunch – my friends, helping me beat this disease. With difficulty, I climb onto the examination bed. It's painful to lie in any position. They never comment on my soreness or thinness. I guess it's what they expect.

"Just relax," he says, as he prods my abdomen. Then, as always, it's, "Right, turn over and we'll just take a look," and I roll over dutifully onto my left side, right leg drawn up for the weekly inspection of my bottom.

The shock of searing pain pinions me to the bed. A full rectal examination is being attempted! My mind can't accept what is happening. There is the shock of pain; that this can be happening; that these caring people could be doing this to me. My eyes screw tight momentarily against the pain and open to meet those of the young doctor – *who is still grinning . . .*

"No!" escapes through teeth clamped so tight they feel they might break.

But the pushing continues and I can't move. I'm trapped against the bed, holding my breath, every muscle clenched to prevent it happening, but only worsening the pain. *And nothing is said . . .*

Eventually, I have to breathe out. Fire rams into me, forcing apart swollen, inflamed flesh; pushing, rotating against the raw tumour. A terrible groan rips out of me. Involuntarily, I mouth, "Bastard!"

And it's over.

"Jolly good!" he says brightly, "it's going already."

How could they do this to me? They knew I would never have allowed an internal examination. They'd planned this before I walked into the room – no – from the beginning of treatment!

My brain is exploding. And he's telling me I can get dressed – *as if nothing has happened.*

My insides are a raging fire. Distraught, I drag myself into a sitting position, take my weight on my hands and balance, head bowed, tears streaming as my body lets me down. But the real crying is hidden inside.

These were my friends. I am desolate.

Nobody moves. Nobody says a word. Their silence seems designed to 'normalise' the situation; to make me feel I have to accept it as a routine part of treatment. I'm shaking uncontrollably and snatching at breaths, but there's no comforting arm around my shoulders. Nothing.

Then comes a whispered, "Sorry". But the summer rain has lost its soft caress. And the disparity threatens my sanity.

How could you do this to me? He must have had to do it . . . Conflict rips at me.

"S'right" squeezes out through clenched teeth. Mustn't let them think they've won. *But you'll never do that again!*

I'm struggling to find answers, reasons, excuses, among the turmoil. *It must have been necessary. They knew I would never agree to it, so they had to do it this way, without warning . . . but if they needed to find out if the treatment was working, why couldn't they use general anaesthetic, or give me another scan . . .? How could they . . .? Why . . .?*

My insides and bottom feel like one open wound. The slightest movement pulls at the rawness. I'm hoping someone will help me down, but still no-one moves. Memorable pain shoots up inside me as I slide off the examination bed. Still shaking and snatching at breaths, I struggle into my clothes and have to hang onto a chair to put on my shoes. Strangely, I feel ashamed for them.

"Any questions?

Damaged Goods

They all knew!
But they said nothing

Nothing prepares me for this onslaught
The shock
The searing pain

My protests ignored, they persist
And *still* they say nothing
They care nothing for my pain, my feelings
The desolation of evaporated trust

Worthless, simply a Thing
I know total degradation
In this room full of people
I am summarily isolated
Vulnerable
And in despair

Jaws clamped, I snatch at breaths
The silent, wracking sobs somehow contained
But coursing tears betray
The futile longing for a comforting hand

Something died in me that day
And now
I feel nothing

The nurse takes me to have radiotherapy. It hurts to walk. The pain goes on burning fiercely for at least twenty minutes. Thoughts chase each other in tightening circles. *If I had been eighty, the shock might have killed me . . . it must have been necessary to do it without warning – to save my life . . . he wouldn't have wanted to do it . . .* I cling to this, but it's not logical – 'does not compute'.

Expediency can't be the reason. I'll be back for treatment to my groin in two weeks' time, so why didn't they wait and give me time to heal?

"I . . . called him a . . . bastard!" I stutter disjointedly, in shock.

"Don't worry," the nurse confides quietly, "plenty of people have called him worse than that."

There's an extra radiotherapy session and consultation on Monday.

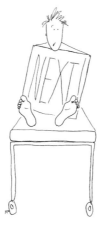

Figure 22.1 Medical might.

I have to face 'Them' again. My insides turn to water as I drive towards the hospital. Eyes downcast, heart pounding, I wait for my name to be called. I'm terrified, but I need them to talk about what happened and explain 'why'.

I've spent the weekend re-living the pain and trauma in every quiet moment. I've cried myself to sleep and woken, crying, to nightmares. Each time the pain and shock are as real as if it's happening right there and then. 'Why?' batters at my head, but there is no answer.

It's my turn. I force myself to enter that room and wait expectantly for words of apology – explanation – comfort. But there's no acknowledgement of what happened.

I don't feel strong enough for confrontation, but I need answers.

"What did you . . . put on your . . . gloves . . . when you . . . did that . . . examination?" The words sound ridiculous. He looks amused.

"I don't remember. KY jelly I expect. Why? Did it sting?"

'Sting'? Why can't they ever acknowledge pain?

"No. It burnt!" *And it wasn't just that!*

But that's the sum total of my protestations! *How could you do that to me . . .? Why did you do that to me . . .?* If only the questions would stream out . . . I need them to know what they've put me through, how I feel. But I can't articulate confusion. I cannot challenge. I am 'Mitzi, Meek and Mild'– an infant needing to protest against a Headmaster. How can I raise the real issue? It's too confrontational. I am too debilitated. I cannot stand the smallest stress. The consultation has moved on, the moment lost once again.

Shut Down
Probe it and prick it
And mark it with 'P'
But you'll never prise out
The essential me

My mind runs in endless circles, trying to find reasons, excuses, to understand the incomprehensible. Somehow, however irrational it is, to make what happened even faintly acceptable, I have to convince myself it must have been necessary – he must have hated having to do that to me.

I know nothing of 'consent',[13] of what they are allowed or not allowed to do to me, but I can no longer play their game. There is nothing, and no-one. The desolation is absolute. I feel detached, wrapped in barbed wire, dead inside.

No-one can see into my head. They can do what is necessary to my body, but they will never know what I am thinking. I have no other defence. As I watch them, watching me, communication becomes virtually one-way, my answers to questions as minimal, my smiles as meaningless and plastic, as theirs. Now *I* make the rules, compliant only to the point of necessity. They had been my team, working *with* me to fight this cancer. Now, I will beat it *despite* them.

Later, I try to tell my GP what happened, but I can't articulate what was done to me – it's too dreadful – it seems too critical of the profession. She reads out a hospital follow-up letter, 'It was impossible to tell if the treatment is having any effect because the examination was so difficult'. The shocking words burn into my head. I write them down, so there can be no mistake. Tears stream down my face. Not because the treatment might not be working. Not even because he'd lied about it 'going already'. But because it seems what they had put me through – and what it has done to me – had been pointless and unnecessary.

DISCUSSION

These poems are particularly raw. Could you have toned down the wording?
Poems can be very emotive. I'm sorry if these are too uncomfortable, but they are a true reflection of my feelings, written at the time. I did not deliberately 'choose' the words. It was therapeutic writing. Feelings took control and 3 am outpourings flowed as if written by someone else.

Was the doctor really gloating?
I suppose the word 'gloating' surfaced because this procedure had been premeditated, and the young doctor was grinning. I'm sure he'd just forgotten to switch off his grin, but the image stayed with me and the effect on me was the same as if he had been enjoying my suffering. But it was a subconscious connection. If I had been asked, I would not have described anyone as 'gloating'.

The presence of onlookers did not protect you?
Their presence made it worse.[28] It felt as if they had ganged up on me – three against one.

Would the presence of an independent chaperone, chosen by you, have helped?
Yes, if they'd had the authority to protect me, but I would not have realised I needed one unless I was told the procedure was going to take place.

You felt ashamed 'for' them?
Yes. They had shamed themselves, not me. I felt degraded, but refused to become their 'victim'.

You had not been asked for consent?
No. Later I discovered that by turning over I had, in the eyes of the medical profession, given 'implied', or 'presumed' consent – a concept unfamiliar to most lay people. Nowadays, such a manner of working would not be tolerated,[29,13] but informed consent was a grey area at that time. This did not lessen the impact upon me.

So this may have been simply routine?
Can using force and disregarding such pain ever be routine? I'm still trying to find a logical reason.

What was the effect of their silence?
I felt trapped into silence.

The procedure did not take long?
True. But the shock, pain and use of force had a lifelong psychological effect.

Did anyone ever explain why they had not waited for you to heal before examining you?
No. What I discovered later only deepened the mystery.

What needed to change?
The need for pain relief should be discussed with patients before any painful procedure.

Patients need to give consent to intimate or painful procedures, however brief,[30] and well in advance of the action.

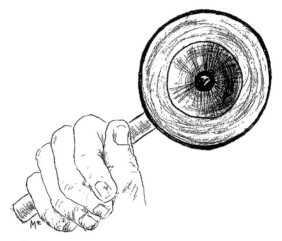

Figure 22.2 Specimen.

The brevity of a painful procedure should not be used to justify lack of pain relief.

Treatment should be about curing the person, not just the tumour.

An imbalance of power, stifles communication. Without honesty there can be little respect and unless patients are respected as people, there can be no compassion.

(In his introduction to *Doctors and Patients: an anthology*,[31] Cecil Helman discusses how the effects of modern data-gathering by diagnostic machines influences some doctors, with 'medical attention focussed on the *body*, rather than the patient' and suggests the resulting abstraction ('paper' patients) can seem more attractive to some doctors than the real thing.)

Chapter 23

'Curiouser and curiouser'[32]
Raging fevers, shaking, aching
Icy, sodden nightclothes cling
I lie in saturated sheets and can't lift the drink that the children bring.
Pain is off the scale and rising,
A toilet roll serves as a gag for biting

And muffles the groans as I bang my head on the wall
　　And tell myself it will all be gone
　　Tomorrow
But, for a week, no GP calls

'Panic' follows the surprise
And "Hospice?"
"No thanks, I'm *going* to get better."
But just now I'm too weak to open my eyes.

The prospect of respite from the 90 mile trek, appeals. I expect to feel under the weather for a few days and tell the children not to worry when I become a little unwell. But the deterioration is rapid and acute.

I like a challenge, but this is ridiculous! The nurse's look of alarm should have warned me of the understatement. I'm burning up, gripped in a terrible fever one minute and shaking uncontrollably with cold the next. I can no longer get dressed. The children leave several half-filled glasses of water by my bed before they go to school, because I cannot lift a full one. *How very strange! I thought very sick people went to hospital, but they have sent me home to be ill.*

Sleep is virtually impossible. My soaking nightgown, taking up the cold night air, clings like an icy shroud as I drag my way to the toilet. The pain of violent spasm is far beyond bearing, yet continues to rise. I can't prevent myself crying, "No! No! No!" But words and head-banging are futile. I clamp my jaws deeper into the toilet roll, hope the flush will drown out the groans and tell myself it must be better tomorrow.

Shaking uncontrollably, clinging to furniture, I stumble back to bed and drag off the nightgown. But the bottom sheet is also wringing wet and freezing cold. I don't have the strength to remove it, so climb naked into bed between the top sheet and blanket. In the morning the children bring a pile of towels so that in future I can lay one over the soaking bottom sheet before climbing back into bed.

'A bit like flu?' Which 'bit'? 'Full blown malaria' would have been nearer the mark. They are the experts. Surely they must know the real effects of their treatments? Why didn't they tell me honestly what would happen? How could they send me home to this?

Kath is shocked at my appearance. I haven't the strength to chat and she does all the talking. She tries to cheer me with some jokes, but it hurts when I laugh. At work next day, she asks the GP to call, but nobody comes. The next day she mentions again that I am very ill and need a visit, but again no-one calls. As I deteriorate further, Kath looks increasingly worried.

"She'll come on Friday, when term time starts," she says, through tight lips. My house is en route to the local prep school which the GP services, but it's the Easter break. Sure enough, on Friday the dogs' manic barking signals a visitor at the back door. I manage to drag myself to the kitchen and stay upright by hanging onto the door handle with both hands. It's the GP all right, but she's brought her 3 year old child along, expecting me to look after her while she visits the school.

It's another surreal moment. For a few seconds I stand there, knees buckling as she chatters, while the floor threatens to swallow me up.

"Gotta lie down", I mumble, interrupting the flow, and stagger away.

"Shall we come too?"

"Don'-mind."

There is no energy left to talk and I'm way beyond the simplest decision-making.

Clutching at furniture, I lurch my way back to bed and collapse. How strange. My eyelids are too heavy to open. It doesn't matter. Nothing matters any more.

She's asking if I'd like a Macmillan nurse.

"Mmmm . . ." It's exhausting to draw breath; a relief to breathe out, 'phut . . . phut . . .' With each exhalation, my chest collapses like a house of cards.

She thinks I'm dying. Never mind, I know I'm not.

DISCUSSION

Why do you think they did not warn you how ill you would be?
They seemed unable to acknowledge the side effects of treatments to themselves, let alone to patients.

How did you feel when side effects became so much more severe than had been predicted?
I felt hoodwinked, naïve, let down. Today's patient information continues to say radiotherapy does not hurt (and it is hurtful to read this) and does not acknowledge possible pain. The effects were so severe, I was unable to think rationally, or deal with my situation.

Why do you think your GP did not call on you for a week?
She probably did not realise the possible effects of treatment. I do not know when she received the follow-up letter I saw later, but it gave no indication that I would need care.

Why do you think they did not keep you in hospital?
Self protection. Out of sight, out of mind.

What needed to change?
Patient information should be explicit and mention expected and potential side effects of radiotherapy.

GPs seem to think patients are under a consultant's care until the end of treatment, while consultants seem to think patients are the GP's responsibility, not only between treatments, but between different parts of a treatment. In reality, they are likely to fall between two stools, with resultant neglect.[33,34]

One caring GP has suggested oncology follow-up letters should be sent to GPs as each phase of active treatment is completed, with details of the tumour, treatments given, expected short and long term side effects, and pathways of care (see Chapter 57).

This information needs to arrive with the GP before the end of each phase of treatment. More use needs to be made of fax and email, prior to ordinary mail. (Secretarial problems can cause delays.)

Patients undergoing aggressive treatment need a specialist nurse/ Macmillan nurse assigned to them routinely from the beginning of treatment, so that palliative nursing care can be accessed swiftly, without guilt.

Chapter 24

Inside Outside
My skin 'don't fit me' any more
It cascades down my frame in folds
Perhaps one day, when I get up
I'll find it crumpled on the floor

Wherever my body touches the bed, it feels as if my bones are trying to push through the skin. Chris, the lovely Macmillan nurse, brings a fleece to lie upon. She also brings warmth, friendship, support and compassion. She suggests I have a rest in the local hospice 'just for a week or two', but I don't want to leave my children. I know I've already turned the corner, even if she thinks I'm going to die.

It's wonderful to have my own Macmillan nurse, but I still have nagging doubts about why I meet the criteria.

"I thought you only looked after dying patients?" I ask, hanging on her words, hoping she will be honest. She says that's a misconception and not everyone who goes into a hospice goes there to die.

The pain has slightly improved by the time I get drugs called 'MST', which is just as well, as they have little effect. My daughter discovers some non-milk-based build-up drinks and I manage small sips throughout the day. During the following week, a community nurse organises a rubber ring to sit on, and other sources of help are drawn in. I'd once been amused when a little boy in local foster care asked me who my social worker was. Now I am going to get one! It's demeaning to be so weak, one of their 'cases', but I'll be grateful if I qualify for a 'Home Help'.

By the end of my 'break', I've regained enough strength to be back on the conveyor belt of hospital visits, drawn there inexorably each day for another two weeks. The area being treated is much smaller than before, just my left groin, and radiotherapy is given from one direction only, so side effects should be less aggressive.

Dead Cert'
'Not 100% sure that the treatment will work'
How I smiled to myself
But I played it your way
Until today

Your loaded questions may have been nifty
But I've known from the start it was 50/50
The odds didn't matter that much, you see
Simply the fact that you kept them from me

I still visit the hospital shop occasionally to get presents for grand-children, but now, surreptitiously, I haul myself up by the banister. One day I bump into one of the ward nurses who asks how my treatment is going. "Over the worst of it now then," she says, when I update her. But at the mention of implants to come, she looks away mumbling, "Oh well, never mind . . . all be worth it in the end," and hurries off. I'm left wondering what she knows. And what I should know.

The Monday and Friday clinic routines continue, but there's no turning over to 'just have a look'. And there's something new in the air. Information is being offered!

"It's not 100% certain the treatment will work, Mitzi."

I don't react, but I'm amused. Of course a cure is not 100% certain! Do I look mentally challenged? Or have I been 'terminal' all along and he is preparing me for death? I don't care what they think. I'm feeling so much better, I'm supremely confident the treatment is working.

So, now, at last, you can offer information – acknowledge possible failure – when it suits you? To prepare me for the inevitable – or so you won't feel bad when I die? Well, I'm way ahead of you. I'm not the one in denial. It's too late to start a meaningful dialogue and too pitiful an offering to persuade me you've had a change of attitude. And far too late for me to believe anything you say.

He doesn't know the GP had told me my chances were fifty-fifty. This scrap of truth is the only certainty I have to hold onto. I smile to myself. Two can play . . . *my* secret. One piece of information *they* do not have – something missing from their mind games.

DISCUSSION

What made your secret so important to you, even though your chance of survival was so low?
They no longer had total control.

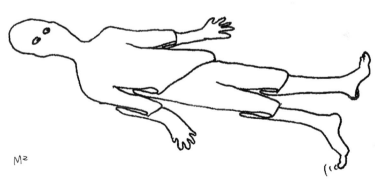

Figure 24.1 Outsize?

Chapter 25

The social worker has a couple of wasted journeys, due to my hospital trips, but finally catches me at home and arrives complete with clipboard and bulging briefcase. He has to see if I meet the criteria for getting help, though he can see how weak and gaunt I am. I can't do anything. I can't even decide what to cook, let alone cook a meal. It's funny how the thought of being able to do the washing up now seems attractive.

"Just thinking about food makes me feel nauseous, and standing up for more than a few moments makes me feel ill," I tell him.

"A bit anorexic?" he queries sympathetically.

'Anorexia nervosa'? Is he saying I'm a bit off my head? Or is there another type of anorexia – without the psychological aspect?

I'm too shocked to protest, but I'm not anorexic! I'm aware that I'm too thin and wish I could eat more. But he's writing something on his clipboard.

It's a great relief to be told I definitely qualify for a home help, but I'm thoroughly disconcerted when he asks, "What arrangements have you made for when you can no longer wash or dress yourself?"

'When', not 'if'!

"But Jimmy!" I protest, "I'm going to get better!"

"Oh! Sorry, Mitzi. Sorry." He steers the conversation onto the date of his next visit, but I'm wondering what is written on his clipboard. *Have they been stringing me along? Am I 'terminal'?*

I've woken in the small hours as usual, but something is different. My drifting thoughts collect and focus. Oh yes! Today Social Services is sending in the cavalry. No support for 8 weeks, but now they pull out all the stops. Sparkle will replace squalor. As my eyes register the accumulated clutter, I realise the carpet is effectively buried. One disadvantage of this bed-sit arrangement is lack of cupboards.

Forcing myself out of bed, I pull on a dressing gown and slowly begin lifting things onto chairs. It's very cold, but too early to have a bath and get dressed, or I'll wake everyone. Even though I move just a few things at a time, I have to sit down frequently to rest. Preparing for the cavalry is wrecking me!

The kitchen is next. As I open the door the dogs charge forwards, sending their water bowl clattering across the room and suddenly the floor is awash. Next moment, five gymnastic kittens launch themselves at my dressing gown, hanging precariously as I paddle unsteadily towards the kettle. I don't reach it. The horse thinks it must be breakfast time and starts thumping his hoof against the stable door. Clearly, starvation is only a matter of minutes away for all.

Coat over nightclothes, feet into icy wellies, I creep outside and manage to drop some hay over the stable door then crawl back to bed, totally drained, but triumphant. The kitchen will have to wait. At least now the Home Help can run the vacuum around my room and do a bit of light dusting.

DISCUSSION

Did you have access to any sickness benefits?
No. I did not qualify for work-related benefits. The social worker said he'd see about getting me something called 'Disability Living Allowance' after 6 months but I thought this meant he expected me to be in a wheelchair by then, so I told him indignantly I was not going to be disabled. He never called back. It was 2 years before I chanced upon information about this benefit and was able to access it, along with a blue parking badge. Later, I discovered that I'd been expected to die within 3 weeks of the GP's visit.

What needed to change?
Seriously ill patients need to be enabled to discuss their prognosis so that they can choose how to utilise their remaining time.[18]

Patients should be offered benefits advice.[35]

Chapter 26 ▬

Time Out
I walk the dogs almost half a mile
Visit sick friends and help them smile
I can soak up summer every day
And watch the meadows turn to hay
Music fills my waking hours
While hosts of gentle, doting flowers
Triumphantly impress, each vying with the rest

I can marvel at swallows slicing by
Watch as bats quarter the evening sky
I can doze under trees or laze in the sun
And I never thought it would be so much fun
And I've so much more to do and see
Now that I'm ill, I am cosseting me

The twenty-third of April, St George's Day and my birthday. A poignant goal. People will be wondering whether I'll reach the next one. Spring is well-advanced. I manage to drag a folding chair-bed into the garden and lie for hours, wrapped in a sleeping bag, watching bees among the apple blossom. The dogs rootle around for a bit, then, pressed hard against my bed, settle into oblivion.

Cancer has helped me to look at life with new eyes: the tracery of branches overhead, the delicious new-born green of emerging leaves. Weeds have become friendly wild flowers, nodding encouragement as a light breeze riffles through them. I doze to the soporific hum of bees and a concerto of birdsong, broken occasionally by squabbling hens.

Suddenly, the dogs start up, barking. My previous boss, the doctor who first asked me to work for the practice, but later sold it, is walking up the drive.

"I'm so sorry, Mitzi". She looks very concerned.

"Why? What's the matter?"

"All this . . . the cancer. I'm so sorry."

I try to reassure her. "Oh! Don't worry. I'm getting better. I'm going to beat it."

She doesn't look convinced.

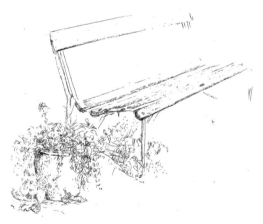

Figure 26.1 Time Out.

"They are saying it's my fault, that I couldn't even diagnose my own staff."

"Who is?"

"That's the story that's being put around."

I'm appalled. "But that's not true!" I exclaim. "You referred me to the hospital. It wasn't your fault that they would not do the barium meal examination. I'll tell everyone the truth and make sure they know it was not your mistake."

It's so kind of her to visit me. She's brought a birthday card, perfume and a lacy petticoat decorated with butterflies and pearls. I am overcome. She had been held in the highest regard by her patients and her absence has been deeply felt.

Mirror, mirror
I look in the mirror, but that's not me
Who is this person that I see?
Her face is falling off her head
And the rest of her droops as if half-way dead

Out with the make-up, on with the paint
Brighten the picture, etch in the faint
Cover the wrinkles of time-worn care
And then just pretend that they aren't there!

The Macmillan nurse has stopped calling. Whenever anyone asks how I am, I say I'm 'fine', because that's what they want to hear. But I'm not. I'm operating on two levels. There's a groove running from wrist to elbow, between radius and ulna, and a bony line dissects my

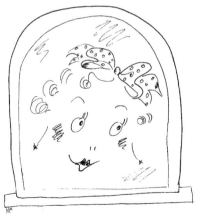

Figure 26.2 Mirror, mirror.

face with its 'witchily' pointed chin. Coping with pain has become a way of life. In the evenings, reptilian in my need for warmth, I stand with my back against the radiator for as long as possible. But now I'm rocking from foot to foot in a strangely compelling rhythmical pattern. Toe/heel, heel/toe repeats the double diamond – like a zoo animal displaying symptoms of stress.

Chapter 27

Indispensable: indigestible
Your expertise: irrefutable
Dedication: indisputable
Eminently suitable
And yet
Immured
And quite immutable

The flip-side, me
Monosyllabic or hypersonic
Practically catatonic
Transmutable
Deletable
Quite simply, unrepeatable

A quivering wreck, red-eyed
Overdriven in overdrive
A trilobite, still full of fight
Yet still without facility
Communication? Out of sight (*My* forte – 'ambiguity')

You'd have more chance of getting it right
With an amenable, erudite troglodyte.

(Conscious of my reduced vocabulary, I was amazed when a friend said my poems contained too many big words, so I reached for a dictionary and wrote this, tongue in cheek.)

The consultant regularly examines my groin lump, but he no longer asks me to turn over. At every consultation, he says, "It's not 100%

certain the treatment will work" and goes on to describe the implant procedure. So much repetition is disconcerting. Perhaps I should be worried. Maybe he doesn't remember what he's already told me, or he's checking my comprehension. Or is it guilt – because he's going to have to do something really horrendous to me?

Sieved!
Breathless

    Emaciated

Withdrawn
    and debilitated

    An empty supermarket trolley
    bullies me with ease

Exhausted
by the
effort of
extracting information and
Drained
    by the
effort of
    trying to please
trying to
make them
believe that I'm coping
When my
s
k
e
l
e
t
a
l
body
    is
buckling
    at
   the
knees

"Mm . . ." is the only acknowledgement I can give that I've heard and understood. He is an expert in his field, so I still have faith in his expertise, even if I can't react when he talks to me. Contained within my fence, I cling to scraps of control. Sadly, I no longer have any expectations of them.

After treatment one day, I stop at a supermarket to buy a four-pack of baked beans for the children. I can't carry it in a basket and a trolley helps to keep me upright, but exhaustion swamps me as I reach the check-out. I wish the trolley was a wheelchair and finish up half lying across it. *I shall have to lie on the floor soon. Fifty pounds for anyone who brings me a chair!* The shy little mouse no longer cares what people think.

Outside the wind has strengthened and presents another challenge. The trolley becomes animated and pits itself wildly against me, propelling me further and further from the car, like a swimmer in a rip-tide. I envisage the headline, *'Supermarket trolley abducts cancer patient'* and am just wondering if I'll finish up back inside the shop when a kind man rescues me.

The slope from car park to hospital has become a mountain. A production line of patients shunts slowly from reception to radiotherapy waiting room, to secondary waiting area, to treatment room and out: peas, thumb-shucked from pod into the waiting world. One day, a child emerges from the treatment room. I know children get cancer, but it's very hard to come face to face with the poor little mite. I would willingly die if he could live. The encounter haunts me.

No-one has told me why the machine treating my groin lymph nodes is different from the one that treated me earlier. The waiting room is tiny, so people are inclined to chat. As I sit here, wishing I could fall asleep, cancer in the bones is mentioned. My ears prick up. *Did the scan show cancer had spread to my bones?*

"I hope you won't mind me asking," I say, but have you all got cancer in your bones?"

"Yes, it's spread to his bones" answers a man's wife, as easily as telling me he likes peanut butter sandwiches. The others smile and nod agreement. Their acceptance is surreal. This place is surreal.

We are all being treated for bone cancer! We are all terminally ill! I have found them out! The shocking confirmation outweighs any sense of achievement.

The gardeners are painting the roses. Soon the Queen of Hearts will appear and shout, "Off with her head!"[32]

When it's my turn for treatment, I ask directly, "This machine is for treating cancer in bones, isn't it?"

The radiographer looks startled, but I need straight answers.

"It's for treating lots of conditions," she replies evasively. Her eyes look away and her words do not reassure. I feel a sense of panic. I need to be able to talk about this, to know the truth. I also need to know why I still feel sick and can't eat and ask when I'll be able to eat properly.

"You should be able to eat properly now." Her evident dismay contributes to my increasing fear. *My insides are full of cancer. How long do I have? Why won't they talk about it?*

She tries to contact a doctor, but it's lunchtime and no-one's available. I go back into this 'waiting room for the dying' and sit alone while she treats the last patient. My head begins to spin. I'm tired of being manipulated and now totally convinced they have been stringing me along. My breathing becomes shallow and rapid. The room begins to go dark. I feel faint and try to open the door, but it's stuck fast. I start smacking my palm against it to make someone hear. The radiotherapist sits me down with my head between my knees and, after a few minutes, I feel better.

"I'm OK now," I tell her, "I can go home now." I'm terrified they will keep me here.

"I can't let you go until a doctor has seen you," she says. But no-one is free, as yet.

"What about your lunch break?"

"That's all right," she says.

But it's not all right. It's my fault she's losing her break.

Eventually, she arranges for us to meet up with a doctor between wards. He thinks my evening restlessness may be due to the sleeping pills and suggests I don't take any more. (Is my body craving more pills? Am I an addict?) When I ask why I can't eat properly, strangely, he asks what I do with my time and I tell him I visit sick friends.

"What's the matter with them?"

The minute I mention someone with anorexia, he responds with a satisfied, "Ah!" and writes on his pad – and I realise my mistake.

"But I'm not anorexic!" Here we go again . . . collecting labels by the cartload.

They let me go and shaky legs deliver me to the car park. I wonder if the radiographer got any lunch. And I still don't understand why I can't eat properly.

DISCUSSION

Why would he have had 'more chance of getting it right with an amenable troglodyte'?
The break-down in communication was my fault. I could not react normally towards them. This should have been a doctor/patient partnership, but we were on different sides, separated by defensive barricades.

Why was it 'sad' that you had no expectations of them?
They were all smiling and pleasant to me and seemed to be trying their best. I still ached to have a good relationship with them, but something had gone.

What needed to change?
Perhaps I needed to be someone else.

Chapter 28

Leaden feet
Sleep calls

The floor yawls

Drawing
me
down

But I make do
    propped
        against
            the
                corridor
                    walls

And I can't walk *there*, any more
I can't sit among *them*
Not again

So you bring me the only available chair
And leaden lids deflect the stares

As I sit, incongruously
Draped
In an armchair
In a corridor
And I could rest here, floating free
Forever

And it's too late now to pretend that I'm strong
So how can I blame them for getting me wrong?

During the second week of this treatment my husband goes abroad for a few weeks' consultancy work, so there's a respite from marital tension.

I've managed the bathing, dressing and driving, but the mountain was nearly too much for me today. I swear it's steeper than before. Somehow, I've made it through the hospital doors and by forcing one foot in front of another, accompanied a nurse through miles of corridors towards the radiotherapy waiting area. But now someone has pulled my plug.

The self-generating, magic porridge pot of a corridor stretches to infinity. Cold and hard as it is, the floor develops a magnetic pull. But I mustn't embarrass the nurse, so I lean against the wall.

"What's the matter?"

How to explain how ill I feel; that my legs can't carry me any more; that the thought of listening to other patients' lurid descriptions of vomiting is too much?

"I . . . can't . . . go . . . there . . ."

"Well, you can't stay here," she says kindly, looking concerned. But my eyes are closing. *I'm sorry to give you a problem. I just need to sleep. Here! Now!*

"It's all . . . those people . . . always . . . talking about . . . being sick."

"Wait here and I'll see if I can get you a chair, so you don't have to sit with them."

People pass in both directions, but I don't look at them. I feel curiously detached. It's taking every ounce of strength to stay on my feet. *They mustn't keep me in hospital.*

"All I could find was an armchair."

How wonderful! She supports me until we reach it and I collapse gratefully, eyes closed, impervious to the curiosity of passing 'traffic'.

Judgement day

They try to lever me out of depression
Assumptions and prodding, are filling this session
So this is support?
Well, I know it's well meant
But the piercing blue eyes stare with too much intent
Trial without jury, no chance of appeal
For it feels like an accusation

How could they rate me so low on their scale?
How could they think that I'd ever fail?
Don't they know I will never give in?
But my body is shaking, I'm weak and I'm thin
My mounting anxiety's manifest
And preconceptions fill in the rest
So they don't get as far as the true realisation

Or wonder 'why'
When I cry

For I'm not depressed, I'm exhausted and stressed
and it's not fear of cancer constricting my chest
       and my self esteem
           just hit
              my knees

AND I'M NOT STRONG ENOUGH TO TAKE CONFRONTATION!

Fragile as thistledown, I'm shown into the consulting room and prepare for the usual 'how-are-you-fine' routine, but instead comes an abrupt challenge.

"Everyone tells me you're very depressed!"

It's like coming up against plate-glass.

"No I'm not!" I retort – a bristling four year old, powerless in the face of adult injustice.

How many more unjust labels will I collect in this place? *I'm not depressed! I'm coping, but stressed! Don't you know the difference? I'm stressed because you decide how much information I need and drip-feed it; because without honesty I have nothing to rely on; because I need to have absolute faith in you – and I can't.*

"It's no good sitting at home feeling sorry for yourself . . ."

I can't believe my ears. How could he think that of me? *I'm supporting other people!*

But I won't justify myself to them. I try to stay strong, but stress is off the scale once again. I'm no match for this onslaught and distraught that they have such a low opinion of me. Salty rivulets of hurt and indignation track down my cheeks, confirming their assumptions, as my body lets me down yet again.

Bright side
Two hours sleep
   (four, if I'm lucky)
Still driving 90 miles a day
Living on determination
   two cream crackers
   and half a yoghurt
     or less than that
And you say
   I'm a 'quivering wreck'
And I think
   'I'm dealing with robots'
But at least *I'm* not fat!

The intense scrutiny has become unbearable. Summoning all my strength, I retaliate, "Well-*you*-don't-help . . . sitting-there-*looking*-at-me!" My eyes snap shut and, in one movement, I spin around so I'm no longer facing him. The ridiculous machine-gun staccato lingers in the silence, to taunt me. I sit here, defiantly clutching at tattered pride, wondering how I can ever open my eyes to face them. It's like being under interrogation again. The relief of closing my eyes outweighs any embarrassment.

"Oh yes! I turn everyone into a quivering wreck!"

He sounds amused. Who can blame him? Part of me wants to laugh with him at my childish tantrum . . . *at this person who is no longer me* . . . Another part cannot bear the hurt. *He thinks I'm a quivering wreck, a coward!* And he hasn't finished yet.

"I could fall under a bus tomorrow . . ."

It feels like a battering. *How ridiculous! How insulting!*

"*I* know that!" My eyes open with the vehemence of my retort.

Leave me alone! Can't you see I need help? But the wail stays locked inside. And the needling continues, less forceful, but still salting the wound.

"We don't want you giving up treatment."

I'm reeling. *How could you think I would ever give in? What do you care? You just want me to continue with treatment on the off-chance you can notch up a rare success.*

There's a long pause, then he asks, "Are you sleeping all right?"

Ah! Insight at last . . .! But I can't let him win. *For me to know and you to find out.*

"I have pills." *But I don't use them.*

Until now, the information battle has been totally one-sided. Now that I've gained a foothold, I'm not about to give ground.

Strung Out

So many things I want to explain
So much I need to say
But the tightness makes me all buttoned and pinched
And the words all get lost on the way

I can hear myself saying such silly things
But you don't know how hard I've tried
I can't open the hidden door
So the meaning stays locked inside

I hear you trying to humour me
I hear you try to be kind
But though I admit I am hanging on
I haven't let go of my mind

This isn't the fear that you think you see
And it's not that I'm depressed
You're just the straw on the camel's back
Something on top of the rest

So many answers I've wanted to know
But I'm snatching at leaves in the wind
Please, just tell me, *without being asked*
And this struggle need never begin

After a weekend at home I feel a little stronger, but have the embarrassment of facing them on Monday for a final check-over. This whole cancer experience is like a character assassination. Somehow I have to make them see past my bodily weakness and recognise my inner strength.

"Sorry about the other day," I mumble with a lop-sided apology of a smile. "It wasn't me." (I'd meant to say 'I wasn't quite myself' but, as usual, it didn't come out as intended.)

"Ha! Who was it then?"

I'm happy to amuse them, but I can't explain.

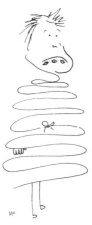

Figure 28.1 Buttoned and pinched.

"A space alien." Might as well match up to their expectations.

And he's writing on his notepad, adding to the list. By the time I leave here, the only label I won't have will be 'religious nut' – and that's probably only a matter of time.

DISCUSSION

Did he really 'needle' you?
That's how it felt at the time – like a barrage of blows – I was so fragile. I felt like a skittle, repeatedly knocked down, hauling myself back up, time after time.

And what do you think now?
He was probably just trying to 'jolly me along'.

You cried, but you were not depressed?
I cried from sheer physical weakness, from exhaustion caused by the treatment, lack of sleep and grinding, ongoing pain. And because I felt bullied.

Why didn't you tell him you could not sleep?
It was an instinctive, childish 'tit for tat' reaction, confiscating their rights because they had withheld mine: clinging to control as a means of defence.

What needed to change?
Patients need someone with communication skills to discover the real reason for their stress.

Hostel accommodation should be available so that cancer patients do not have to travel long distances.

Chapter 29

The Friday clinic brings me to the brink of my second two-week break. The lymph node lump is definitely smaller. When he's finished prodding my abdomen, I sit up quickly and move to get dressed.

"I'm afraid we're going to have to do another rectal examination."

I can't believe you said that! I want to shake the words away. It's another mind battering. Even if they are blind to the psychological damage caused earlier, they must realise the physical pain that examination had caused. And they know deceit won't work twice. They're not aware that I know it had been pointless, that they'd lied about it. They don't know I have been suffering relentless playback.

Has this, too, been planned from the beginning? Why aren't you offering general anaesthetic? I'll agree to anything if you control the pain.

My mind is struggling to absorb the shock. ". . . afraid . . . can't . . . say 'yes' . . . to that," I stammer.

"We need to know the size of the tumour to estimate how much wire to order."

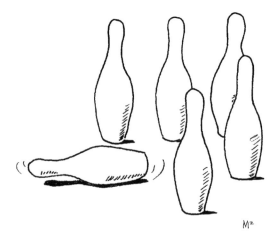

Figure 29.1 Skittles.

Why couldn't I have just said 'no'?

"It's very expensive wire."

My pain versus their expense! *Then offer me pain relief!* Even now, I'm hoping they will find redemption. I feel trapped and prepare to do battle if they rush me.

But there's only silence. And I'm Alice,[32] shrinking fast again. My pain means nothing to them. I mean nothing to them. I feel utterly worthless.

Silence hangs like a fire curtain between us.

Don't try to make me feel guilty. I'm valued less than a piece of wire. But what price your self-respect?

DISCUSSION

How did you feel when you were told they needed to do another rectal examination?
I felt profoundly shocked and doubly worthless.

What needed to change?
Before treatment begins, patients should be advised what procedures it will entail, so they can discuss the need for pain relief.[30]

Chapter 30 ▬

Implant time, and the last lap. I'm in a side room because of the radiation risk. It's at the far end of a men's ward. It must be the only vacant single room. A TV stares blankly from one high corner, but the remote's been mislaid. There's an en-suite shower, but a plastic sign on the loo warns 'out of order'.

"I don't know why that's there," says the nurse, testing the flush. "Anyway, if you have any problems, let me know."

"What else could I use?"

"You'd have to use a bed-pan – or the toilets at the other end of the ward."

'. . . *other end of the ward'?* I'd never make it in time – and imagine the agony of trying to balance over a bedpan . . . When I find the leak in the pan, I keep quiet.

I'm nervous, but thinking positive. At home last night, in my husband's absence and the relief of separation, I realised I could no longer live with him. Anything had to be better than this, for both of us. As I removed my wedding ring, a weight lifted. Somehow, when I'm strong enough, I'll break free.

It's good to have my own room. I pretend I'm in a luxury hotel until a foul tasting laxative they give me shatters my daydreams. I ate little food yesterday, but nothing today (the thought of going to the loo when there are wires in my backside is terrifying) so the irritant produces plenty of pain and blood, but little else. Next morning, the nurse brings a second dose. My insides and bottom feel raw.

I've brought books and sewing to combat boredom and am busy hemming a skirt when the consultant drops by. "I know it's a first time for you, but implants are my forte," he preens.

Yes, you're an expert and I'm lucky you'll be doing it. You will look after me, won't you? But, I'm tongue-tied and can't reply.

Music spills suddenly from my tape-recorder, startling us both.

"How did you do that?" He looks bemused.

It's a home-recording. There was a gap between songs. Will 'bewitched' be added to my labels?

The long afternoon is punctuated only by occasional visits from the tea-lady and a nurse. Day-time television is irritating, but I can't reach the controls; evening TV is better, but the volume climbs unchecked. A nurse rescues me from the din as the ward prepares for the night. I lie awake for hours, wondering what the next day has in store.

Very early next morning, just as I'm just sitting up in bed, the door bursts open and six people pour through, filling this tiny room: the oncologist, four other men in white coats and a nurse. I'm so shocked by the intrusion, my heels dig into the mattress and in one instinctive movement I shoot backwards, until my back presses against the bed-head. Six pairs of eyes are trained on me. I feel a fool. I can't look at them, only glance at each as he introduces them in jocular fashion. I notice one has a turban.

"Doctor W has come all the way from India to *see* you," he beams. "Doctor X has come all the way from Singapore to *see* you . . ." He continues in the same manner, introducing each foreign doctor in turn, enjoying his little joke. I smile, dutifully.

My heart's thumping and I can hardly breathe. I suppose it must be an unusual technique and they have come to watch so they can help patients in their own countries. They whisk out of the room as fast as they'd arrived. I'm left dazed, tense and on my guard against further invasion.

The procedure is to be done tonight. *(The only vacant theatre slot, or after the late night movie on TV? Must keep my sense of humour under control . . .)* Apprehension grows during the long day. In the

108

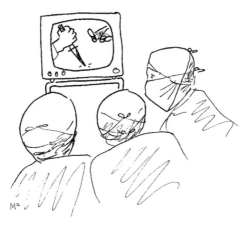

Figure 30.1 Late night movie.

afternoon an anaesthetist calls in and mentions that he's a replacement. He doesn't smile once. I can't help wondering if he resents being called in to work unsociable hours. It's rather unnerving.

After what feels like a pre-sacrificial weighing, he surprises me by saying, "I understand you're feeling nervous about these implants." More statement than question, the cold delivery holds no reassurance.

"No I'm not," I smile and add good humouredly, "but from the way everyone keeps going on about them, I'm beginning to wonder if I should be worried!" I'm just trying to break the ice.

Big mistake! There's not a twitch of a smile. I'm being friendly, but does he think I'm mocking them? *(Am I impossible to please – resenting false smiles, but dissatisfied when there are none?)*

"In that case you won't need a pre-med," he states firmly, closing the option.

I thought patients always had pre-meds before operations, but feel obliged to rise to the challenge. Wishing I had the nerve to back down, I reply, "All right then, I won't", and add, "just as long as I wake up again". My brother died on the operating table.

"Oh, you'll wake up all right!"

But did I imagine that edge to the tone? Perhaps my fear is being misread as antagonism. Anxiety increases as the evening drags on. The nurse turns off the television around 10 o'clock. "They'll be coming to collect you soon," she says. And leaves.

The ward closes down for the night and I'm left alone, my only companion the hammering in my head. And silence. Confidence wanes; anxiety becomes fear. I'm trying to control my breathing. *I wish I had someone with me. I wish I could have a pre-med.*

After an endless three quarters of an hour, a trolley clatters in with the shocking impact of an executioner's arrival and they wheel me out. We stop in an ante-room and my heart's racing as they start the anaesthetic injection. For a moment, I contemplate flippancy, 'I'm going out and I may be some time . . .' but there's no warmth in their eyes.

"Shall I count to ten?" I smile uncertainly, still hopeful of some friendly response.

"Can if you like."

I sink into blankness, feeling very, very alone.

DISCUSSION

Why did you press yourself against the bed-head?
I was very frail and it was a reflex, defensive movement. I felt shocked, outnumbered, overpowered. A specimen.

Did you mind that four doctors had come to watch the implant procedure?
No, although it was a little embarrassing to think of them all looking at my bottom.

What needed to change?
Patients should be asked their permission in advance when a group of clinicians intends a bedside visit.

Pre-medication should be offered to people undergoing surgery and painful procedures (including day-case patients undergoing major procedures).[36]

Patients should be offered information about pain relief before procedures are carried out.[37]

Chapter 31

When we're through
Night casts a skein of velvet dreams
As talons rip
And consciousness screams.

And it was no time at all
for her, for him.
For me, it stretched interminably.

"That's it!" *(That's it!)*
At last hope grew
But flared and died, relief short-lived
"One done."
And five more still to do.

I'm in my room, but there is no pain. Haven't they done it? The silence of the night envelops me. Yes, it's all over. I'm lying on my right side and someone is doing something to my backside.

"What's the time?" I ask thickly.

But as the nurse replies, I'm gripped with indescribable pain and realise the anal canal muscle with six wires threaded through it is going into spasm. I struggle to keep quiet, but a primeval groan is wrenched from me. As the pain subsides, I turn my head for help. But there's no consultant, just a nurse and the turbaned doctor, seen so briefly this morning. He's trying to connect the implant wires to the radioactive source, but he keeps sighing and 'tutting' and I realise he can't do it. He completely ignores my groans.

"Not long now", says the nurse, brightly, flashing a smile. I grit my teeth, expecting him to finish any minute, thinking she means the pain won't come again.

"We'll give you a painkilling injection when we're through."

'When we're through'?

Another contraction. Once again, I'm gritting my teeth so hard they might break. Obscene pain . . . animal noises. My noises . . .

I feel ashamed. *But why don't they stop the pain?*

"Nearly done," she says. And I believe her. *Any second now it will all be over!*

But the 'tutting' and sighing goes on – as does the agony.

"Nearly done," she keeps saying. "Nearly there."

Must hang on . . .

At last, she cries, "That's it!"

He's finished! It's over! She's going to give me an injection! The relief is so great I want to weep.

"One done, "she says, reassuringly. "Just five more to go . . ."

The remaining connections are gradually completed as the doctor gets the hang of how to do it. Only then does morphine bring blessed oblivion.

"Let us know the moment you feel any pain begin," emphasises the nurse next morning, as she gives me another injection. "Don't wait until it takes a hold."

So, by the time the consultant arrives I'm lying on my side, pain free and comfortable. He walks around the bed, looking very pleased with himself. I'm waiting for him to talk about what happened, to say 'sorry'. I'm in terror of that pain. *Tell me you won't let it come again.* He smiles and says everything went very well and he mustn't stay long because of the radiation, but he'll call again tomorrow.

Doesn't he know about the pain? Hasn't the nurse told him the other doctor couldn't do the connection? Why didn't they warn me about the pain? Was the procedure purposely done late at night so that other patients would not hear my groans?

My mind cannot accept that they could knowingly put me through this. *Why weren't you there? You said implants were 'your forte', so I thought you would be doing it.*

Crazily, I wonder if there is some medical reason why pain relief cannot be given during implant connections – I need to justify the lack of humanity. Is this just another issue no-one can discuss because it's too uncomfortable – for them?

The next sixty hours pass with little discomfort and virtually no pain, although I'm extremely apprehensive when two nurses come to remove the implant contraption.

But, that day at least, it's the nurses who get the shock. As they pull back the sheets their eyes meet in shared alarm.

"Oh! – Just a minute, you've bled a little," they say. But I've turned enough to see their faces and glimpse the pool of blood in the bed. So that's unusual?

The removal procedure is pain-free. All I feel is relief. It's hard to come to terms with the disparity between what I suffered earlier and the high level of pain control that followed.

DISCUSSION

You did not realise that doctors learning the technique would be actively involved in your care?
No, I had no idea.

Why do you think it took so long to complete the connection procedure?
Later, I learned that the doctor had been told what to do while in theatre, but was practising it for the first time. The ordeal lasted about forty-five minutes.

What was the effect of the nurse's encouragement?
It gave me false hope and caused me to endure lengthy, unacceptable pain.

Why didn't you tell the consultant about the pain?
I did not feel able to confront. Also, I did not know if it was something I was expected bear.

But he might have been unaware of what had happened?
Yes.

What needed to change?
Patients' suffering needs to be acknowledged if there is to be change.
   Patients' permission needs to be obtained before doctors learning a technique (effectively 'students') are actively involved in their care.
   Nurses need to be empowered to speak out without fear of reprisals.
   Doctors practising new techniques need adequate supervision.
   Levels of pain relief differ from country to country – foreign doctors' practice must meet UK standards.[38]

Chapter 32

The consultant sends me home with the words, "I'm afraid you are going to be a bit sore."

Hmm. Just like I was 'a bit' ill after 4 weeks treatment? I'd been more than 'a bit sore' when I first presented to my GP and pain has increased daily since then. I wonder why he bothers to say something so banal.

Incredibly, pain shoots up beyond anything I have endured and keeps rising. At the first sign of needing to defecate, the pain becomes so acute it makes me swear and stamp my foot as I make my way to the toilet. I'm seriously head-banging and repeating "No! No!" but the pain is relentless. Afterwards I collapse, crying on the toilet floor.

The pain increases each day and is so bad I think I must be over the worst, so it's days before I allow myself to phone the busy Macmillan nurse, Chris. By then I'm living in continual anticipation of the next day's torture, unable to think rationally.

And now the playback is two-pronged.

I feel guilty for taking her from dying patients and I'm so ashamed at not coping with the pain, I convince her it's not urgent. So it's another twenty-four hours of hell before she arrives.

She bustles in and begins, "You've been having some . . .?" But I interrupt wildly, "Would-you-like-a-drink?"

She looks perplexed and tries again, gently. "Mm, yes, please. But you've been having some . . ."

"Coffee-or-tea?" I cut in again, the very air sparking agitation. Anything to stop her saying that word.

She searches my face and I know she's reading terror in my eyes. On her third attempt, I collapse onto a chair, distraught, pleading with her not to say the word that forces me to re-live the agony.

Next minute, she's kneeling at my feet, grasping both my hands. And I'm rocking backwards and forwards and experiencing the pain all over again.

She's lovely, but she doesn't seem to have any idea what the treatment has done to my insides, or why I'm in so much pain. "Sometimes a small piece of haemorrhoid can get trapped and the pain is cruel," she says. "Shall I take a look?"

Does she think anal cancer affects just the anus? I tell her she wouldn't be able to see anything. Apart from pain down my left side and in my groin, and the soreness and fragility of my skin inside and out, my main tumour site is now a 4cm wound, well out of sight, affecting a quarter of the circumference of the anal canal and penetrating down into the muscle. *Hasn't anyone told her about the effects of treatments – of my particular treatment?*

She contacts the oncologist who says there shouldn't be this level of pain – unless it's an ulcer. *'Shouldn't be'? That figures!* The surgeon who delivered the original diagnosis offers to fit a temporary colostomy. I am almost tempted, but how can I let them near me?

It takes days to sort out the pain. MST is totally ineffective but, finally, short-acting Palfium (dextramoramide 5mg) does the trick – as long as I get the timing right. Chris tells me I should use it before defecation, that's at least 3 times a day. But when I try to get a second prescription from my GP she says it's an opiate derivative and I should take only one pill a day.

So I have to ration myself! And suffer. The anticipation of knowing the drugs will run out at the weekend adds mental suffering to physical torture. The pain is so bad I feel like a mad dog, ready to bite at anything to relieve it. I am in terror of that pain and, once again, feel abandoned. I cannot endure any more. That night I contemplate driving to the railway crossing at the end of the village and ending it all.

The GP finally relents, but sends a written prescription with Kath, rather than the actual drugs. To make absolutely sure of getting them, I have to drive twelve miles to the chemist, every bump in the road ripping me apart, and stand swaying in a queue, the aching rawness consuming me as I struggle to prevent myself falling over.

"How do you feel?" asks the Macmillan nurse next day.
And I mutter, "Broken."

DISCUSSION

What did 'a bit sore' mean to you?
It meant they could not acknowledge pain, or the effects of treatment.

Why do you use the word 'torture'?
It's not a word to be found in many medical journals, but having daily, off-the-scale pain, and knowing it will come repeatedly in the days ahead, has the same effect as torture.

What needed to change?
Potential and anticipated side effects of treatments need to be acknowledged.

Patients being treated according to clinical trial protocols should either be kept in hospital, or closely monitored at home.

Improved communication is necessary between tertiary and primary care.[39]

Macmillan nurses' instructions to patients regarding drug dosages should not be over-ridden by GPs.

'Your pain is the breaking of the shell
That encloses your understanding'
And
'Even the stone of the fruit must break
That its heart may stand in the sun
So must you know pain'
From 'The Prophet', Kahlil Gibran

PART II

Chapter 33

Lucky Patient 10,003
Doctor, with a capital 'D'
Thanks for the treatment
Thank you for 'me'
Job well done, praise well earned
"Effusive thanks to all concerned"
Thank you for succeeding with me
Doctor, with a capital 'D'

So you worked your best magic
Waved the right wand
Made the wayward cells respond
Lucky patient, with a capital 'P'
But where's the *person* who is me?

I have emerged with a survivor's gratitude, but a teenager's resent-
ment – and all the guilt this jumble of feelings engenders.

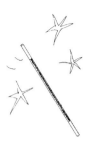

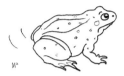

Figure 33.1 Wrong magic?

Discrepancies and anomalies gnaw away at me. Kindness versus barbarity. Nightmares and replay continue to plague me, invading my head in every quiet moment. Each time, I re-live the shock and pain. Each time, it's as if I am hoping to change the past.

The need for answers has become an obsession. Why was it done that way? How could they send me home to be so ill, without support, to pain that left me suicidal? Why didn't anyone acknowledge the side effects that could happen and ensure relief was in place? Why didn't they talk to one another? Why had no-one cared? How can I be feeling like this, when all I should be feeling is gratitude?

For some time now, I've not only been making repetitive patterns with my heels and toes, but rhythmically chomping my teeth together. Even when I'm aware of it, I don't stop. I need to do it. Perhaps it's a comfort reflex, like thumb-sucking. When my first check-up looms, just one month after the end of treatment, I'm too weak and in far too much pain to risk a rectal examination. Chris attends instead and explains my absence. I can only wonder at how little they seem to understand the effects of their treatment.

Whoops!
Love skips
Love slips
Love trips
Love lies bleeding, love lies

Love sighs
Love cries

Love tries
Resignedly, love dies

A week later my husband flies back from abroad. I am still too weak to stand for more than a few minutes, still have constant, dragging pain, immense pain on defecation, acute faecal urgency and eating and sleeping problems. I'm very frail and over-sensitive to noise. Frequent hot flushes hit me with the severity of sun-stroke and, despite feeling the cold dreadfully, I have to run icy tap water over my arms and head for relief. My lower abdomen feels like a volcano. To make it bearable, I wrap a bag of frozen peas in a tea-towel, and stuff it into my knickers.

It's a painful twenty mile drive to collect him from the station. As we pull out into the busy afternoon traffic, his first words etch themselves on my brain.

"Are you back at work?"

He has no concept of my suffering. Perhaps he hasn't noticed I'm skin and bone. 'Dressed and driving' equals 'well enough to work'.

"No, I'm not back at work." And I'll never go back to that surgery. What is left of my life is my time.

Later that day he tries again, adding "Well, all I know is, there's more money going out than there is coming in."

He just doesn't understand. Our finances are something he will have to deal with. I have enough to do just fighting cancer. And it's time to face facts. He needs to recognise that our marriage is over. I let him know I'll be leaving as soon as I'm strong enough. Living within a broken marriage is destroying both of us.

"You can't afford to leave me," he says, not unkindly. I think he's stunned. But I have reached the point when I am ready to sleep on the streets . . .

Aware that the marital split will affect more than immediate family, and full of guilt for upsetting them, I ring my husbands' siblings to warn them of the impending divorce. My own parents and brother are dead and now I'll be cutting myself adrift from this extended family. Our lives, and our children's lives, have intertwined. We share holiday memories of sand mazes, dune surfing and cold North Devon winds. Apologising profusely, and a little 'off my head' with Palfium, I wail down the phone, "I just can't take any more". Goodness knows what they think of this mad woman.

A couple of weeks later my employer stuns me by asking when I'll be returning to work. "Give it a try", she insists. "Just come in for a couple of hours."

I can't rush. Getting to work on time is stressful. The soft car seat pulls at my sore insides. When I arrive at the surgery the telephone screeches a greeting and continues to jar my nerves every few minutes. The repetitive high pitched squeal of the computer modem is unbearable. Patients' exclamations of, 'I thought you were dead!' become amusingly predictable. I manage to work alongside Kath for an hour until the need to lie down is overwhelming.

"You'll never be as good as you were before!" predicts my GP.

No? I'll be better, stronger! I've been walking the dogs a little further each day, willing one foot in front of the other, but progress is frustratingly slow. My employer is happy to sign me off. "I can't go on paying you. You understand, Mitzi?"

No severance pay. I've worked for her for a year and for the previous doctor at that practice for about 5 years. Maybe something should be due to me, but I feel too debilitated even to think about pursuing this. When I'd pointed out that the recent pay rise had not been included in my pay packet following diagnosis, I'd been told I was lucky to get anything. But money means nothing to me now. People's acquisitiveness appals me. However, if ever I am to leave my husband I will need to earn enough to keep my son as well as myself and that means getting a good reference.

I contact a government 'back-to-work' scheme, hoping to access training for a worthwhile career, but they won't see me for just an hour or so and I'm not well enough to attend one of their all-day assessment sessions.

A trip to town should be a treat, but by the time I have driven there, I'm drained and feel a sort of panic need to get back home and lie down. In a nightmare version of musical chairs, I have to be ever mindful of the nearest toilet's location. The pain of imminent need is excruciating as my bowels stretch like a water-filled balloon and it's difficult to stand up straight as cramps take hold. Managing the unmanageable becomes part of life. I can't help wondering whether some of these problems are due to my flesh being torn unnecessarily during the protracted implant connections.

Another hospital check-up. How simple that sounds; how difficult to drag my feet here, every muscle tensed. It's only by convincing myself that I won't let him do a rectal examination that I manage to attend. But some challenges are unforeseen.

"Are you back at work?" he asks. Soft words, scalpel-sharp. He cannot know the connotations or their impact. I can understand he'd like me to be back at work – as proof that his treatment is effective and harmless. But I can't tick his box.

When he has examined my abdomen, I sit up quickly and tell him

I'll let him know if the tumour returns. Spoken aloud, the words sound ridiculous. He smiles.

"I know you're special and it's a very pretty skirt," he cajoles, gently, "but I can't have any idea if the treatment is working unless I can examine you properly."

Why am I special? Because I was expected to die? Pretty skirt? Don't treat me as if I'm an idiot.

I'm pressured between the need for his expertise and fear of allowing him to do what I'd sworn he'd never have the chance to do again.

"You can't know, Mitzi," he coaxes.

"I will know." But conviction falters.

He's right, of course. I have so much pain, it's impossible to tell whether or not it's due to cancer returning. I can't let it come back and take hold or I will have gone through all that for nothing. No alternative then. Reluctantly, I face the wall, curled and foetal, and reach out instinctively to clasp the pillow to my chest; a child seeking security from her doll.

It hurts, but the pain isn't fierce like last time when I was unprepared, resisting and raw. But, like once before, a tear has collected in the corner of one eye.

I'm 'doing very well', apparently. Because I've survived this long? Nothing clever in that.

"In fact, I'm very pleased with myself," he adds, with a proprietorial air.

'What about me?' cries the 3 year old. *'Who is pleased with me?'* Childishly, I resent his self-congratulation. Who will acknowledge what I've been through? *What about the unspoken – the unspeakable?*

"We don't want you waiting so long another time," (smile).

One more unjust label to hurt and demoralise me. I should be pleased when he says there's no sign of cancer. But I don't care. I feel nothing.

DISCUSSION

Why didn't you care about being clear of cancer?
Constant playback was affecting me far more than fear of cancer. In any case, I could no longer believe anything they said.

What needed to change?
I needed more than they could give. I needed them to care.

Chapter 34 ━━━

Against the Grain
You cannot care, cannot afford to care
Too many passing this way
A daily tide that would engulf and drain
Just part of the job to smile, to show concern
Pretend to feelings that you dare not feel

Being here
Makes me acutely conscious of the essential sham
Sometimes I play along
Sometimes I buck against the rein
The masquerade
The habit worn
The wretched game

Just a name among thousands, am I
Less than a bird-blink
Less than a fly's foot on the wall
When I am here
Simply a tumour; treatment; prognosis;
One of 'them'

Being here makes me feel
I mean nothing at all

And you –
You cannot afford to care
But, those of you who do,
I hear your pain

Surprisingly, when treatment ends, part of me misses the daily contact and I feel even more isolated from society. The days stretch emptily; fatigue is so limiting. I have no stamina and no role. I am 'the cat that walks by itself'.[40] Plenty of time for navel-gazing. I rest in the garden and slowly, painfully walk the dogs, trying to unpick the conflict in my head. 'Sucked in, chewed up and spat out' – that's how I feel. A battered, brutalised child. I know I'm an emotional wreck, grateful for the treatment, but screwed up. So much, so wrong, yet they all seem to think they are doing it right! Isn't that sad?

"And nobody knows, tiddley-pom . . ."[41] I try to push it all away and concentrate on gathering strength to leave my husband.

But I'm still on the merry-go-round of monthly check-ups. Even when these stretch to bi-monthly, the stress of facing 'Them' does not lessen: drag myself back, go through the motions, smile, submit; pretend things never happened. And, in between, continue to suffer the nightmares, playback and pain.

I'm still a patient, a compliant thing, chained by necessity, defined by my appointment schedule, the bungee-elastic reeling me in, affirming control. Announcing my name, and that of the doctor I have come to see, categorises me; the designated seating area proclaims my cancer label. When my name rings out I join the lepers, shunted along to the next humiliating public identification.

Of course I fear cancer returning, but I can deal with that. It's being a patient that's so difficult. Now I cannot bear any level of control. Even the daily dose of disgusting Lactulose syrup, enslaves me. My ragged nerves wince at 'How-are-you-fine', while 'Are-you-back-at-work?' reduces me to a shrinking 'thing'. Then comes the examination. And I'm worthless again. Even as the consultation ends, anticipation of the next begins.

DISCUSSION

Pretend what 'never happened'?
The events that haunted me, the replay.

How could taking Lactulose syrup be 'enslavement'?
Having to take it daily, to comply, meant they were still controlling me.

What needed to change?
I needed counselling, but I did not realise it at the time.
  I needed to communicate my feelings to them.
  Patients and health professionals need to talk to one another.

Chapter 35 ▬▬

Beyond

The blackness of deep space can hold no fear
For one who catapulted round the sun
Slipped through Time Warps with relative ease
Played marbles with Red Dwarves and 'tripped'
Down wormholes of disease. This one,
Who trampolined the Time-Space Continuum
Sapped energy from pulsars and scattered pennies down black holes
For fun.

I have lain there looking at the cup, too heavy for the wasted arms.
Dessicated. Lips desperate to sup
Eyelids shuttering, energy spent
Seared by pain in a different dimension, an unknown plane
Outside comprehension.
In another time, my universe tilted
Balance shifted, impaired
Now $Q - A = Uncertainty^2$

Resolve has hardened like sun-warmed wings
But emergence prompts bombardment
From unfamiliar things: strange extra senses, blowing my mind
And supercharged synapses, powered by solar wind
Offer interplanetary flight

There is a ragged tear in the fabric of space
Reaching beyond Relativity.
New life spawned
Ancient Order scorned by haemorrhagic, unencumbered thought
Well able to transcend this worldly place.

I have known the beauty of deep space
Joined the dots and fashioned neural networks from the stars
Ranged through galaxies without end
Caught wayward comets in jars
Seen the Dark Side, bathed in Titan's pools and dropped back
Changed.

Privileged. Awareness-honed
I stand outside this game.
With an astronaut's perception, I can feel the pulsing earth
Know the value of a leaf
And mock the girth of self-inflated man.

I live in an exclusion zone.
Yes, I crossed swords with cancer
But I've mutated and grown.

My gratitude to the staff who saved my life is bottomless (no pun intended). But the cancer experience does not end with treatment. Everything has altered. My perspectives. My values. Me. It is difficult to describe adequately my sense of feeling 'different'. Being close to death has given me an enhanced appreciation of life that must surely be unattainable by any other means. The impact of the experience has been so immense, I feel irrevocably changed, like a member of a privileged group – a race apart – an astronaut who has learned the 'meaning of life' and returned from the stars.

DISCUSSION

Was anything else significantly different about you?
Yes. I had lost my inhibitions, and that was empowering. But I was torn by conflict, I'd learned not to trust and I couldn't watch films containing abuse.

Chapter 36

Redundant, but free
Life is a gateau, a trifle for tea
(Eat it up, slurp it up, greedily!)
Loved every minute that I've wallowed in it
But the rest of the pudding is for me, me, me!

The children have learned to fend for themselves. It's probably character-building, but I feel I'm letting them down. As wife and mother, I have been the care-giver. Illness has taught me to accept help, graciously, to look at my own needs. I have had to learn to be a little selfish.

Life is incredibly precious and this is *my* time. Fun time! What do I want to do with the rest of my life? It has to have meaning. I want to help people, but I'm too old to be a nurse. I'm too fragile to cope with domestic chores, let alone full time work. Treatment seems to have affected my body's ability to regulate temperature. I learn to keep a hot water bottle and blanket on the settee, because after a few minutes of inactivity, I start shivering violently. Yet the mildest sunshine burns my knees and the heat of overhead spotlights in shops is as fierce as an electric fire too close to my head. My comfort zone is very narrow.

Painting was my favourite subject at school. If only I could have gone to art college . . . In the autumn I enrol for deaf-signing, adult literacy teaching and life drawing classes. I also sign up for a 10 week course at the local dry ski slope. *I am invincible!*

Not invincible enough. After impressing the tutor on my first day, I progress from nursery to main slope, but wasted muscles and pain in my groin from radiotherapy-damaged lymph nodes make it impossible to maintain the pigeon-toed 'plough' position in which the skis act as brakes. Two bad ski falls and then a riding accident leave me unable to push, pull, lift or carry without acute pain in my shoulders, neck, back and head. Carrying Christmas shopping is particularly difficult and I have to go through shop doorways backwards. Eventual physiotherapy for my shoulders exacerbates neck pain and my head pain becomes excruciating as soon as I put on the surgical collar I've been given to wear at night. Only sleeping pills bring relief. I cannot use a pillow. When they discharge me, saying they can't do any more, my whole body is still locked in spasm.

Debility forces me to waste precious time, but I push myself to the limit and complete and pass the deaf signing and adult literacy teaching courses "Slow down, Mitzi," friends advise. *Why, when I'm enjoying myself?* But I have to lie down for an hour before dragging myself off to teach adult literacy in the evenings and eventually see sense. Helping one of the clients privately at weekends softens the guilt when I resign.

If I am to leave my husband I must find full time work. In my youth I had been a London secretary, but my shorthand is rusty, I have no computer skills and no desire to write other people's letters for half their pay. I need something more creative, fulfilling and worthwhile. At an eventual back-to-work assessment, I'm advised to update my secretarial skills and keep art for a hobby. It's not what I want, but I duly attend college under a government scheme. On the first day, a picture of a filing cabinet is projected onto a screen and a mimsy-pimsy voice asks, "Can anyone tell me what this is?"

I close my ears and spend half an hour filling in job applications before leaving the class, secure in the certain knowledge that secretarial updating is not for me. The next batch of assessments and re-assessments is 6 weeks away, so I fill in time by brushing up my French in the college language laboratory.

At the next interview, my ambition to help people leads to a place on a Royal Society of Arts Counselling Skills course and a corresponding placement with Age Concern. For the next year I'm very happy, visiting elderly people in their homes three days a week and assessing their needs. The level of responsibility and trust placed in me is so high, it's like being self employed. However, as well as having continuing fatigue and lower body pain, the juddering of the old car's heavy diesel engine makes my shoulders, back and neck feel on fire. Various pills are either ineffective or cause excruciating constipation.

Outcast
Why did I turn from your tender kiss, the peck upon the cheek?
Why was it more than I could bear?
Why so hard to speak?
Because I felt unworthy
Untouchable
Unclean
The moment held such poignancy
For a leper of so many moons
You cared enough to plant a kiss
Upon this wrinkled prune

I crave human touch like a deprived child, like that monkey someone reared experimentally without animal or human contact. Yet when a colleague attempts a perfunctory 'goodnight' kiss on my cheek, I shy away like a virgin!

"I only meant . . ."

"I know. I know. Sorry."

I'm so closed up within myself, I can't react normally. It's impossible to explain and I drive away quickly to end the embarrassment.

Chapter 37

Two-monthly check-ups progress to 4 monthly. Home circumstances become increasingly bleak, the need to move out ever more urgent, job applications ever more frantic. Hopes are raised and dashed with a succession of interviews. I write a good letter, but once we reach the stage of, 'why did you leave your last position?' smiles and questions become syrupy. They slide in 'How frequent are your hospital check-ups now?' as they share knowing glances, and wrap things up as soon as is seemly.

I've had my turn. You're more likely to get cancer than me! But I can't blame them. My face droops as if I've had a stroke. Debility and pain win in the end and I resign myself to the prospect of living on state benefits.

The check-ups grind on relentlessly. I wonder when they'll become an annual event and for how long they'll continue, but when I ask what is planned, I'm told simply,

"We'll see how you go on."

Why can't he tell me? Is he expecting it to come back? They never weigh me or take blood. Why don't they give me another CT scan? Am I too old? Not worth the money spent?

"How do you know the cancer has all gone?" *And hasn't spread microscopically?*

"You'd be in trouble by now if it hadn't," he says, cryptically.

So it's still my pain versus your expense. *You're happy to wait until I double up in agony one day. That's nice.*

"If it comes back, when and where is it that likely to be?" *What should I be looking out for?*

"We don't know."

But, again, the hesitation had been noticeable. (Later I discovered research had already shown the most likely site would be at or near the primary site.)

"I want to know all that you know," I say, hoping he's feeling expansive. But that 'teacher knows best' smile is the only reply.

"Are-you-back-at-work" hits the spot with heightened effect and this time he throws in another gut-wrencher.

"Things settled down at home?"

Thoroughly nonplussed, I'm instantly transported into the black hole that is my marital state. I had not expected such personal probing. The question assumes a salvageable home situation, when it's long been past crisis point. I'm rigid with stress. *Does he think we have just had a tiff? How can I possibly reply to that?*

"Don't want to answer?" he breaks in. So completely off-track.

"Can't . . . do anything . . . 'til my son's . . . taken his exams." The words stumble out.

"Which exams?"

What does it matter, 'which exams'!

DISCUSSION

What needed to change?

Patients need to be treated as adults, to be 'kept in the loop', told what symptoms to look out for[42] and encouraged to report them.

Exploration of personal issues is best left to appropriately qualified counsellors who have time to give support.

Chapter 38

The counselling course teaches us not to be judgemental, to listen, hear and accept. We learn how to support people in crisis, how to enable them to talk about their fears. We are taught to combine detachment with empathy (offer a branch, not jump into the pond). Good practice must ensure there is no 'ownership of the client', no fostered dependency, no feeding our own 'need to be needed'. The ability to admit when we are out of our depth and help clients access other agencies is essential. If only doctors and nurses were taught all this!

The tutor's exercise this morning is to see ourselves as others see us. Several people describe me as 'serene'. There's a surprise! But the resolve to break free from my marriage gives me a veneer of serenity.

We explore each other's key words.

"What does 'cancer' mean to you?"

"Pain and isolation."

"What does 'patient' mean to you?"

"Degradation; humiliation; stress; conflict; being controlled."

There's no stemming the tears. That's how they learn about the cracks and the papering-over. That's how they learn about the poems. And that's how I learn I still have a long road to travel.

Vinegar and Brown Paper
Ode to my poems
You are the phone that never rang
You are the song I never sang
You are the footstep on the stair
You are the friend no longer there

You are the book I never wrote
You are the words I never spoke
You are the painting locked inside
You are the tears I had to hide

You are the hurt I could not vent
You are the force that lay unspent
You are the load I had to bear
You are the pain I could not share

You are the passion in my soul
You are the salve to make me whole
You are the dreams that haunt me, still
You are the need I now fulfil

I never set out to write poetry or to use writing as a therapy, but conflict and playback did not diminish with time. One night I'd gathered together my notes about things that did not add up, to prove that their 'game' was not all in my mind, and in writing down how each event had made me feel, I'd slipped inadvertently into 'poetry mode'. After that, poems began erupting regularly, night after night around 3.00 am. They were simply a release of repressed feelings as my need to communicate what was so wrong spilt over. I didn't consider them to be real poetry. I called them my 'pomes'.

Writing them had helped me to sort things in my head. The tutor said they deserved to be shared, but who would want to read them? I'd shown the first few to a friend. "But Mitzi" she'd said, aghast, "that was over a year ago!"

"No," I'd replied. "That's when it all began."

Chapter 39

Relay Race
It was a gleaning time
It was a moment lost
It was a catch of breath
A blink, a nothingness
Nor day, nor night
Nor yet twilight
A second's glow
Enchantment in the air
And there was no-one there, but me

A baton dropped between the sun and moon
A momentary lull
A chance to join the fun and hand it on
Before the race swept by again

The light took on a fantasy
The sigh of wind had dropped away
And not a creature dared to move
Especially not me

And I knew a magic moment when the moon stood still
As the moon came laughing over the hill
So I snatched a magic moment
And I caught a magic moment
And I held a magic moment
When Time itself stood still

As I walk the dogs slowly down the lane one evening, I feel at
one with nature, a minute part of this wonderful world. One day
my bones will feed the cycle of growth and beauty. And that's
fine.

When the counselling course ends, I'm amazed to be accepted
onto a 4-year part-time Foundation Diploma Fine Art Course.
I'm going to be an art student! Summer is spent doing art-course

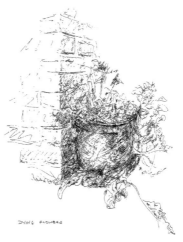

Figure 39.1 Homework – dying flowers.

homework. Making that first mark in a new sketchbook gives me the same buzz I'd felt as a child.

In September, a nurse colleague from the counselling course recruits me to help set up a cancer support group. She sees me as a success story, useful for boosting clinicians' and patients' morale. It's a little uncomfortable to be a trophy, but I'm happy to help. She asks me to contact the national charities, CancerLink (later merged with Macmillan Cancer Support) and BACUP (British Association of Cancer United Patients – now Cancerbackup) who provide us with sets of patient information booklets on various cancers and treatments. What a pity no-one told me about these organisations when I was first diagnosed.

At the opening meeting, a demarcation line is drawn between 'them' and 'us' when we are asked to identify ourselves as 'patient' or 'professional' and say what we want from the group. The Chair and Vice Chair (hospital social workers) are definitely in charge and seem to expect people to want to talk about their experiences. I can't talk about what happened to me. It would frighten other patients who might then refuse treatment. But in any case, I cannot articulate what happened, even to myself. Most people want information and to talk to others in a similar situation. I try to establish that I'm there to help.

The Vice Chair puts up a flip-chart and lists the different emotional stages that cancer patients will experience: denial, anger, bargaining, depression and, lastly, acceptance.[43] There is a stunned silence from patients and carers. Not only has acceptance of death been included as an inevitable part of the cancer journey, but to discover that what we should be feeling and when we should be feeling it has been predetermined is even worse. I can't relate to this, any more than I could to the assumption that I would think 'Why me?' at diagnosis. I've only experienced 'Their' denial. And why should the diagnosis of cancer make me angry? – I certainly would not blame doctors if they could not cure it. My acceptance of death came at the beginning of treatment and I had no wish to bargain. Depression? They haven't mentioned the stress and conflict of being treated like a mental retard! *Allow me to know what I think and feel, even if it differs from the rule books.*

The wife of a seriously ill patient bursts into tears and rushes out of the room. I follow to comfort her. She feels as I do. They seem to have a need to categorise, to neatly package, to control. Who has decided these things? Have they had cancer? Time for cancer patients to re-write the text books! Ever afterwards, I have an aversion to flip-charts.

DISCUSSION

The poems expressed what you had not been able to communicate to healthcare staff?
Yes. Things that could not be said at the time. Some things were taboo.

'Taboo'?
Questions seemed to signal 'inability to cope' rather than 'need to know'. Raising uncomfortable issues seemed to question clinical competence (their possible 'failure'). Anomalies built up. I found myself keeping quiet, not only to show I could cope, but also to 'protect' clinicians.

You felt strongly about the list of emotional stages people experience?
Some cancer patients may go through these stages, but I had not.

How did it make you feel?
It reinforced the feeling that, by becoming a cancer patient, I had lost my autonomy.

You did not feel anger?
No. Why should I? I could not believe that some patients became angry with clinicians who gave them the bad news. A cancer charity originally planned to publish one of my poems (Damaged Goods) alongside an article on anger, until I told them it was supposed to express devastation. I wished I could have felt anger. It might have been healthier.

(In 1997, following a diagnosis of breast cancer, the breast care nurse greeted me in funereal tones. "It's a dreadful time."

"Actually, after a 5-month wait for a referral, it's a relief," I told her, "but very inconvenient and frustrating." By then I was doing a degree and working frantically to prepare artwork for an assessment and end of year show.

"Frustration can be very close to anger . . ." she returned, glibly.

Aargh! In that moment I very nearly felt the anger she seemed determined I would feel.)

People read into things what they expect to see. Perhaps much of the 'anger' seen in cancer patients is due to expectation. Perhaps most anger is generated when information is withheld.

What needed to change?
It was inappropriate to confront patients with the list.
Patients' feelings need to be acknowledged.
Please – no assumptions. They hurt!

Chapter 40

The oncologist has always given me plenty of time to ask questions (getting adequate answers has been more difficult) but never asks about specific side effects of treatment. The ubiquitous smiles and constant bonhomie, along with my indebtedness and need to endure, combine to gag me. GPs don't seem to know anything about cancer treatments or their long term effects. I feel I am left to cope alone.

'Once a cancer patient, always a patient' I'd read somewhere. After treatment, it seems that people imagine every little twinge is cancer returning. Delay and you're stupid; mention symptoms and you're a hypochondriac. When I find the breast lump, I monitor it for two months, trapped by pride. The GP confirms it's not just my imagination and refers me to the oncologist.

"I don't think it is anything," he says "but we'll get a mammogram, just to make sure," adding as he makes for the door, "but if it is, it's nothing to do with this!"

'*Nothing to do with this?*' Sounds like 'It wasn't me! It wasn't me!' Why should I think there's a connection with anal cancer? Is there something else I should know?

The mammography machine is a recently installed facility. A woman who has recently undergone surgery for breast cancer is called in ahead of me and a few minutes later her piercing screams make my hair stand on end.

"Oh! That's cruel!" she sobs. My turn next.

The mammogram shows nothing, but the experience is so painful I swear I'll never have another.

(Years later, when I found mammography too painful following breast cancer treatments, a kindly radiographer explained she could increase the machine's pressure slowly to keep within bearable limits. This way she was still able to obtain useful images without leaving patients traumatised.)

DISCUSSION

What do you think was meant by 'it's nothing to do with this?'
He was probably reassuring me that the original cancer hadn't spread. But the message that seemed most important was that he had not failed.

The mammogram was too painful?
A year later, the department admitted the machine had been set to maximum compression – unnecessarily. They apologised and promised it would not be so painful another time. I could not believe them, so declined further invitations.

What needed to change?
Cancer clinicians should be offered regular counselling[18] to help them deal with 'failure' and loss. This would facilitate openness and enable them to discuss 'difficult' issues with patients more easily.

Radiographers' training should remind them of their duty to discuss and minimise pain and raise awareness that, especially following surgery or other treatments, a patient is likely to be more susceptible to feeling pain.

Patients invited to mammography need to be informed that pressure can be adjusted according to a patient's tolerance of pain.

(More openness in written patient information might improve take-up for the national breast-screening programme.[44])

Chapter 41

Watershed
I hear you calling me across your counterpane
And know a sudden pang
A childhood memory
The scrap of silk against my cheek to comfort me

In lapis green I dive beneath your quilt
And revel in your wilderness, your freedom

Spreadeagled upon silken sheets
Steeped in luminosity
I mould my body to your curves
Drifting at the edge of sleep
Threaded to infinity.

Sea-wife am I
We merge as one
Another life begun

Hammock me in liquid jade
Lull me as I swing
Comfort me with your viscosity
Smooth my cheek
Ease my pain away
Let me stay, let me stay

I float on mirrored clouds and let exhaustion flow
An albatross
Thermal high, in effortless flight
I seek no landing place
Here is there peace for me at last
Your vast warmth to poultice me and buffeted only by the waves

I give myself completely to your mood
Tiny patsy in a giant's paw
Once close your jaw and I am sand

But vent your rage upon some distant shore
Cherish and succour me
Let be

Rocked and gentled, cradled in your arms, I surge and flow
And listen at the keyhole of your world
And see a myriad lives unfold.
A thousand lullabies are sung
Wistful, haunting melodies, to help me cry
For I must learn to weep if I would know the luxury of sleep
But so hard to let go

I hear the Divers of the Deep expectantly calling
Inviting me, enticing
Willing me to join their Company
And I can feel the pull of silken strands
Silken shrouds entwining
So easy it would be, to slip and slide, down, down
Hair streamering
Seaweed tangling a crown
Brown wrack my wrap
And soft green filaments fashioning a gown
So easy, so easy
Nor yet a wave to buffet me
Entombed

But what use life, if bland?
I need the sting, I need to walk the edge
To taste the spice, to dare
No tomb, no shroud, no winding-sheet for me!
At last the tears can flow
And slumbering monsters of the icy Deep are washed
Their sleep unchecked and my release unknown
But dreams, re-drawn, are filled with summer snow

Precocious wavelets slap and tickle, urging me to play
Some sulk and go skittering away
And so I spend the day in endless leisure
I skip and chase the infants of my sea, finding my peace
In children lies my pleasure.
Their laughter is my salve, my therapy
And in their innocence, my sweet release

And now, rare privilege bestowed

You lift your coverlet
And let me peep upon your secret treasure
Gold-dust filters through my hair
Diamonds and emeralds dazzle there.
Camouflaged, these jewels lie
Disguised from mortal eyes, where limpets cling
Once dried upon the shore they are but ordinary stones and gleam no more

But nothing lasts forever
I turn for one last, cherished memory
And find the blue has 'run' into the green
The faded canopy has drifted down to meet your tattered quilt
And moondust spilt across the silk

I'd visualised myself floating in warm seas while practising relaxation, but it's not until the next year that I'm well enough to travel and enjoy the real thing. Family friends let me use their flat in the Algarve. My son brings a friend and Kath comes with me to enjoy the treat.

The sea is so buoyant I can float with arms and legs completely relaxed. As I flop to and fro with the movement of the waves, the physical pain is soothed away and with it some of the emotional trauma. At some point, I must return and deal with the difficult times ahead, but for the moment I can let go.

Chapter 42

Country Mouse
Hazy, in the summer
In the summer, in the city
Sitting pretty (lots of cash to stash)
Before the buzz begins
Before the full fairground swings

I sit and stare at gilded chimney-pots
Tower blocks
Concrete blocks

From my box they squat
On plots where trees could stretch
And mesh with sky, please the eye
Without imagination-stretch

Why must planners' eyes see only rectangle, diagonal
Soulless dimensional jungle, tangle
Wretchedly, without imagination?
What a lot of rush and tear, not getting anywhere
The come-and-go; the traffic flow
Nothing still, except the traffic-jam
Still, here I am
Still here

And how am I supposed to call this 'life', and 'living'
When all is alien to my very being?

My eyes, unseeing, know again the solace of the dew
The morning-light
The hedgerow-slanted view of life
The call of crows

A squall of crows takes fright, a handful flung against the blue
Blank page bespattering, yattering
Black tatters hung askew
To flap and remonstrate, to castigate
In honeysuckle-heavy air
Heady air

The screech of brakes breaks reverie
Within my box I sit and contemplate my lot.
Getting late
Not yet too late for me
With second sight
I know this can't be right

My daughter has left college and accepted a job as designer for a top ski-wear company and moved to London. How will she, a country mouse, survive enforced city life, I wonder? When I leave my husband I will be impoverished. Will I, too, be forced to live in town, so that amenities are within walking distance?

Her current horse is an eventer, young, boisterous and huge (16.3 hands high). Even with an extra loop of rope over his nose, I'm not strong enough to control him and one evening as I'm bringing him in for the night, he barges through the gate, knocking me to the ground. I close my eyes as hooves flash above me and momentarily wonder wryly if I've gone through all the cancer treatments only to die from a kick to the head, but somehow he manages to avoid trampling me. He has to be sent away on loan and is later sold. Although we could not have kept him once I'd left here, it's a great wrench and I feel I've failed my daughter.

Walking the dogs around our fields becomes ever more poignant. How I love this place, yet I have to let it go. The dogs bounce around me, happily unaware of the betrayal ahead.

Initiating divorce proceedings is not easy. The emotional and physical strain of breaking up a thirty year marriage is greater than anticipated, the burden of guilt high, even though I'm convinced it's in everyone's best interests. The kindly solicitor who eased me through will-making now deals competently with my request.

My son has to decide which parent to live with, his dilemma worsened for both of us by my uncertain future. It would be dreadful if he chose to come with me, but cancer came back.

In order to find out my real chances of survival, I write to BACUP, agonising over the wording, desperate to convince them I'm capable of coping with the worst news. The openness of their reply is the first acceptance of my 'right to know' and my competence to cope. It's a huge boost to my morale. It seems in order to get an indication of my prognosis I need something called my 'TNM staging' (just one more thing no-one has thought to mention) and they've enclosed the formula for working this out, according to how far cancer had spread at diagnosis. T stands for tumour, N is for nodes and M for metastases. But the next check-up and opportunity for questions is 3 months away. An eternity.

Week after week, I tramp between estate agents and the Citizens Advice Bureau. For the best chance of getting my own Income Support I need to apply after I've moved out of the house, but Housing Benefit will only be paid to applicants already claiming Income Support, and only paid in full if the rent is regarded as 'reasonable' according to the numbers of bedrooms and inhabitants. How many bedrooms will I need? Will my son be coming with me? How will I ever manage to leave my husband?

Chapter 43

As the November hospital appointment draws near, all thoughts focus like rays through a magnifying glass. So much depends on being able to prise the truth out of Them. This time I must win!

I'm shown into the consultation room but, after a wait, the nurse pops her head around the door to apologise, "Sorry. The doctor's been delayed."

"It doesn't matter."

But my insides are churning. At least I am not waiting half nude. After reading an excellent article, 'With Your Clothes On', which described the effects of 'therapeutic deception' on the author and how she narrowed the gap between her doctors and herself,[45] I started emulating her by leaving my pants on during discussions with consultants, to raise awareness of patient dignity. Minutes tick by, stress mounts, every muscle a hawser – and still no consultant. The nurse comes to apologise again. Perhaps there's an emergency among terminally ill patients upstairs. I feel sorry for him.

When the door bursts open, it's not my consultant, but someone I've never seen before. I'm shocked and disappointed. Only my oncologist is familiar enough with the tumour to know whether or not it has returned. The nurse knew the oncologist wasn't here. Duped again. Should I refuse to let him examine me? But I've shrunk to 'just-a-patient' status.

"Get those . . . things off and turn over!" he sputters peremptorily, indicating my pants.

No social niceties then. None of the usual friendly chat. Speechless and intimidated, I pull off my pants and lie down. For three months I've been steeling myself to be assertive enough to get vital staging information. Now I'm faltering at the first post.

A quick, rough examination follows. I feel like a lump of meat. He consults his notes.

"That's eighteen months. You've done very well." And he's turning away!

"Four months!" he barks, as he makes for the door.

It's now or never . . .

"I have a question." I force out the words, breathless, but resolute.

"What?" He stops in his tracks; the nurse is wide-eyed and wary.

"I have a question," I repeat, with difficulty, pressing home the advantage.

I'm struggling to breathe, but my eyes lock onto his, ready for any deviation from the truth.

"I need my TNM staging." Somehow, I must be assertive. Getting this information is crucial.

"What?" Wrong-footed, he's getting louder.

"My T – N – M – staging," I enunciate quietly, my gaze pinning him in surprising role reversal. No disrespect intended, but I'm drawing on my stubborn streak. For my son's sake, I must not be fobbed off this time.

He looks through my medical records and reads what I already know, "The tumour was 4cm with inguinal node involvement."

I'd pointed out the inguinal node lump in the first place! Why can't he admit to further spread? What about the two places I saw on the scan and the pelvic pain that had kept me awake at night? *There must be something in my records warning him not to tell me any more.*

"And the rest . . .?" I encourage. *You're running late. I'm sorry, but I've waited so long and I need to know . . .*

He flips through my file again in growing impatience and says, sharply, "There's nothing else. What makes you think there were any more?"

"I saw it on the scan!" But I'm clinging to cobwebs as my breathing lets me down.

"You 'saw it on the scan'?" he repeats in disbelief, flashing a jaundiced look.

"There were at least two more places."

He delves into the records again.

"There was 'possible involvement in the mesenteric region, but it was impossible to tell, because the treatment had started already'," he rattles off, tetchily. "If there were any more they must have been on another scan."

There was definite involvement! I still feel the pain! Why won't he even confirm things I already know about? I'm losing another battle.

"I only had one scan." It's so hard to be assertive when your body wants to crumple.

"Well, there's nothing else!" – tersely now. "You have a right to this information, but I can't give it to you." Then, out of patience, he closes the file and rounds on me derisorily, "Anyway, what's the matter with you? You had this cancer, you've been cured. You never-even-had-an-operation! Why don't you go out and enjoy life?"

I go cold. Thoroughly shaken and no match for this confrontation, I struggle to clamp down tears. He turns away. All hope of discovering my prognosis is receding.

"Four months!" he barks again – the imperative flung over his shoulder as he makes for the door.

"Oh! I don't think so," I mutter grimly through tightened jaws. I will not be seen by this gentleman again.

I'd had to park the car streets away from the hospital. Shocked looks from passers-by barely register as I stumble along, wild eyes streaming, face contorted in despair. Reason suggests otherwise, but it really feels as if they are trying to drive me out of my mind. Half blinded by tears, I drive back to college and, helpless to stop the flow, sit rocking back and forth in the car for what is left of the afternoon.

Why are they purposely withholding information? Am I paranoid? Do mad people know they are mad? Don't they know what harm they do? 'Forgive them for they know not . . .'

I'm hanging by a thread and I know it. Obstinacy kicks in. I won't let them push me over the edge. That evening, I write to the oncologist for my TNM staging.

My letter is returned with T2 N2 M0 handwritten across it. According to the staging formula and the scan showing spread to both sides of my pelvis, it should be N3. He's minimising again, tailoring the truth to protect me. My GP is my last hope. She has to convince him that I really need to know!

She looks at the TNM figures in disbelief. "Did he write that?"

"Well, I certainly didn't!"

She seems stunned and checks his signature against earlier correspondence, then she reads out the letter from the hospital doctor who had upset me. ". . . Her primary tumour was 4cm long, the node in the left groin was 1.5cm and there was involvement of obturator group of nodes on the left side. Considering the stage of the disease at the time of treatment, I think she has done very well." "However," she continues, "since she continues to worry about things which a usual patient would not, it appears to me that maybe she has some thyroid problem. I did not have the courage to suggest it to her but if you agree with me maybe you would like to investigate her thyroid function."

We both laugh aloud. My questioning had been persistent, but I'm amazed that he had actually feared me! Me – Mitzi Mouse! (The thyroid test later comes back negative.)

Then she looks sideways at me and delivers a bombshell.

"Of course, you know you are T4?"

So she has not been open with me after all. That sounds terminal – but I think she's got it wrong. From the staging formula sent to me, 4 centimetres does not mean T4 when staging this particular cancer.

She asks me to write down what information I want and she will send it to the oncologist with a covering letter. I ask how many cancerous sites there were, extra to the main one; whether they were they all in lymph nodes (medical terms for sites please); what size they were; whether he has treated anyone else with as many involved sites and if so, whether they are still alive. He surely can't be mistaken about my need to know this time, even if I am struggling with medical terminology.

His reply says my staging was T2 N1 M0. He says he has 'treated other patients with similar extent of disease who have remained alive and well, but equally, there are others who have not been so fortunate'. *Meaningless!* 'The chances of recurrence are greatest within the first 18 months . . .' –*Why couldn't they have told me this earlier? What else haven't they told me?* He also says enlargement of adjacent external iliac nodes makes their involvement likely, but not certain.

So now it's 'N1'. At this rate, soon I won't have had cancer at all! At least this is more proof the dumbing down has not been all in my mind. I list all nodes that have been mentioned as affected, or possibly affected: inguinal, obturator, mesenteric region and external iliac. Maybe the obturator or external iliac nodes are in the 'mesenteric region'. I wish I knew.

The GP at first refuses to give me a copy of the letter on the grounds that it is 'his letter', but I know patients have recently been given the right to access their records. She asks me to put a request in writing. I have come prepared with paper and pen and she caves in. She also gives me copies of earlier correspondence, from which I glean: 'carcinoma anal canal; L posterior quadrant 3–6 o'clock, extending 4 centimetres. 2 nodes palpable L inguinal region – malignant'. I send the information off to Cancerbackup.

DISCUSSION

How did you feel about the doctor's remark that you hadn't even had an operation etcetera?
It was inappropriate and hurtful, but probably due to his busy workload.

What did the comment about your 'unusual worrying' mean to you?
It confirmed that they attributed my stressed appearance to fear of cancer.

Weren't you afraid cancer would return?
Yes, but I was determined not to let the thought mar what time I had left.

How did you feel when your GP received a different version of your staging?
Vindicated.

And when you learned details of potentially affected lymph nodes?
It was a start, but I wanted complete answers.

What needed to change?
Patients should not have to struggle to fit information together.
  Patients should be offered information about their prognosis routinely. Those who do not want it could decline.

Chapter 44

Two weeks later, I secure a lease on a two bed-roomed bungalow in town and my son decides to come with me. We'll just hope for the best.

Christmas fast approaches. And my daughter's birthday, 3 days later. To preserve some semblance of normality, I plan to move most belongings into the bungalow, but remain sleeping in the old home until New Year's Eve. It's crazy and illogical, but I can't make sensible decisions and I don't know what else to do.

Possessions mean little to me now. The division of spoils has already been agreed, the packing done under a watchful eye. Lifting boxes into the car causes days of excruciating back and neck pain.

Christmas passes in a welter of forced smiles, misery and anticipation. On the thirty-first of December, 1991, almost 2 years after diagnosis, my daughter returns to London, my son and I leave home – and I apply for state benefits. As I pass through the kitchen for the last time, the dogs huddle together dejectedly beneath the table. So far, I've managed to ignore their silent pleading, but as I carry the last boxes to the car, it's time to face the accusation in their eyes. Whoever coined the term 'hang-dog' got it right.

"Good dogs. See you soon." The promise to reclaim them one day is built on nothing but hope.

Next morning, the hum of traffic nudges me into consciousness. I've done it! A temporary home for my new, and perhaps temporary, life. The aftershocks will come, but for the moment relief is amazing – although the mattress is hard as asphalt and my bones feel pulverized. As I try to move, pain shoots through my head, neck and shoulders. Lifting my head between my hands, I turn onto my side, tip out of bed and scramble over boxes to start my first day of freedom.

By pure chance, the bungalow lies conveniently close to college, and is also outside the 3-mile radius from my son's school, which means his travel costs will be reimbursed. Money from a small legacy has covered the deposit and will pay three months' rent, but I've no idea whether I'll be able to afford household bills. If I don't get state benefits soon, will bailiffs take my few possessions? Will Social Services declare me 'unfit' and remove my son?

I soon learn to re-use tea-bags and in the evenings sit shivering, wrapped in a duvet, in front of the half lit gas fire. My son seems warm enough.

BACUP replies swiftly to my enquiry. I rip at the envelope and my eyes devour the words: 'With anal cancer, the presence of secondary cancer in the inguinal nodes can give a five year survival rate between 15% and 25%'. *Yes! Yes! Yes!* My chances are not great, but at last someone is treating me as a competent adult, entrusting me with empowering, information. I literally jump up and down for joy. Only someone who has been disempowered to a similar degree could ever understand what such honesty means to me at this moment.

I scan faster and faster: "This figure would include people who had not responded well to treatment . . ." (so the chances of cure could be better) "and is not predictive of what will happen to any one individual . . . published figures . . . inevitably out of date."

I wonder what is so significant about the fifth year.

DISCUSSION

You welcomed bad news?
The news was secondary. Someone recognised my right to full, independent information. And I could believe it.

Chapter 45

How-are-you-fine!
Help me overcome my sadness
Please ignore the traitor tear
Offer me some love and comfort
Spare a moment of your time
Like a child, deprived and battered
I so need a hand in mine

Apart from the usual pain, two places within my abdomen feel raw. Reluctantly, I tell the GP and three days later I'm being seen by the oncologist. I've heard there is now a new 'counselling' nurse and I'm hopeful she will help me get information.

"Show me where it hurts," asks the consultant as I prod around ineffectually, trying to find the tender spots, but it's difficult to locate small, deep-seated areas of soreness in wobbly guts, especially under scrutiny. I prod deeper.

"Huh! Anything will hurt if you dig hard enough!"

He's smiling broadly at his own humour. So is she. This is worse than before. Now there are two of them to mock me.

He prods my abdomen, now a taut drum, but doesn't locate the sore spots.

"Probably pulled muscles," he concludes.

I haven't pulled any muscles. They share the joke. I'm the time-wasting cancer patient, running true to form. I wish the floor would swallow me up.

Stressed to the eyeballs, I'm waiting for him to ask me about the abortive encounter with that other doctor, but he doesn't refer to it. Instead he consults his clip-board and mutters, "Let's see. When is your next appointment . . .?"

"I don't know. I tore it up." The shocking words are out before I can stop them. *Might as well be hanged for a . . .* I seem to be set on 'self-destruct', but I need the chance to counter that doctor's version of events.

Ripping it up had been imbecilic, uncharacteristic, but the only outlet for my feelings *People who feel they have no voice do things they would otherwise not do.* I'd let the appointments clerk know I could not attend, so the slot would not be wasted.

"You-tore-it-up?" he echoes, eyebrows raised, smile broadening.

I'm perversely pleased to note his incredulity. It makes a change from him shocking me.

I need you to know how dreadful that encounter had been. I need your support. This is all going horribly wrong.

"Yes." *Ask me why!*

But, as if not to be denied his fun, he begins again, "Now, when is your next appointment due . . . Oh yes! I almost forgot . . . you're *never . . . ever . . .* coming here again." It feels as if he's taunting me. A child showing off to a classmate.

Am I supposed to have said that – in that childish tone of voice? What has that horrid doctor told you?

I straighten my back, straining to breathe. "I won't see – that – doctor – again." The words jerk out quietly, shredded dignity gathered in – childish missiles my only ammunition.

"Probably pulled muscles," he repeats decisively. Then finally, "Are you back at work?" hammers the last peg home.

"No." I have no intention of going back to work at that surgery. And no intention of telling them this – or what I *am* doing.

An appointment will be sent. And I'm left alone with the nurse counsellor, holding myself together with difficulty and aching for two years' overdue support.

"I see you have 4 children," she begins, glancing at my notes. "Are they all still at home?"

"No." But that doesn't mean I'm sitting at home feeling sorry for myself. My children are well-travelled, independent. I've long since learned to let go.

"Husband still at home?"

Disappointment replaces hope. They know something about my home circumstances. They have my new address.

"No!" Hackles are rising. I can see the way this is going. Sure enough, she delivers the final salvo.

"Plenty of time on your hands, dear?"

Where is the empathic approach, the open questions? What sort of counselling training has this nurse 'counsellor' ever had?

A withering look is enough. She retreats, leaving me to get dressed.

DISCUSSION

You tore up the appointment card?
Outrage and frustration at the memory of the consultation with that other doctor had boiled over when the appointment card arrived.

Why did you admit to bizarre behaviour?
It was spontaneous. Perhaps adrenalin acts as a truth drug. I was too weak to deal with this stressful situation.

Yet you seemed to want to provoke him?
He seemed to want to provoke me! I felt defiant, pushed into defensiveness. I was fighting to gain some control of the consultation, but I could hardly breathe. It felt like 2 against 1.

What needed to change?
I needed an advocate.

Chapter 46

Memorised?
Scrutinised
Itemised
Categorised
Patronised
Dehumanised
Disenfranchised
Institutionalised
Randomised?
And filed
But not yet finalised

A month passes and still I have no income. The Benefits Office says, because I am doing a part-time college course, my case (*I am another 'case'*) has to go before an adjudicator – which could take months!

After moving house, I'd registered with a new GP. He's young and gives me lots of time, but when I try to tell him about the traumas and the ongoing playback I'm still experiencing, he says, "I've had cancer".

I shut up then. My experience is too much for anyone, too uncomfortable, too challenging. I don't want to lay blame. In deepening conflict, I am torn between the need to speak out to change things for future patients and reluctance to criticise those who had once been kind friends. Who had saved my life.

I'd hoped for 1 year of life, and already I have had 2. The approach of spring brings the next hospital check-up. I dread facing the consultant and nurse 'counsellor' so much, I postpone the appointment but, as before, leave plenty of time for another patient to be seen in my place. Two weeks later, I return home from college to find a new appointment on the mat. I read it twice. According to the date and time, I should have been at the hospital that very morning! The letter has a first class stamp, but I can't make out the date of posting. I telephone immediately to make my apologies (although it's not my fault) and explain what has happened. Getting through to the right department takes patience and costs precious money.

When the next hospital envelope drops on the mat, my insides turn to water, but it's not a new appointment. It says they understand I hate attending for check-ups, so they will not be sending any more appointments. If I have a problem, I can contact them. They have discharged me! I try to console myself that at least now there can be no more withheld information, no more nasty surprises. But I feel cast adrift.

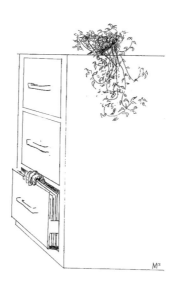

Figure 46.1 Filed.

DISCUSSION

The post did not arrive before you left for college?
The single delivery always came at lunchtime. Years later I read in my medical notes: 'she *says* the post arrived after she had left home'.

How did this make you feel?
It was all part of not being heard, of judging me by their standards.

'Their standards'?
Their standards of honesty.

How did you feel when you were discharged?
Abandoned. I needed them as a safety net. I also needed to maintain contact if I was to have any hope of resolving issues and effecting change for future patients.

Why were future patients' needs so important to you?
I needed peace of mind. I wasn't 'hearing voices', but the need to prevent other patients suffering what had happened to me was a permanent, leaden conscience. Sometimes, when events replayed in my head, I found myself protesting aloud – even in public! That was frightening. I thought I was going mad.

What needed to change?
Medical notes should afford patients the respect health professionals would like for themselves.

  Discharge plans should be discussed with, and agreed by, patients.

Chapter 47

"So you've had cancer?"

"Yes."

"And you're doing a part-time art course?"

"Yes."

I'm going through divorce proceedings, but it feels as if I am on trial.

Minutes earlier, for what had seemed an eternity, I'd sat motionless on a bench in the dismal, windowless inner lobby of the Divorce Court, nervously expecting my husband to arrive at any moment. Sharing this space had been a couple who looked as if they had slept in their clothes. Occasionally, they bellowed at two grimy children scrapping on the floor, faces and sleeves encrusted with snot. Lawyers in black gowns had appeared intermittently, consulted the blackboard on the wall behind me and disappeared, my presence unacknowledged, even by a glance. The sign, 'Bailiff's Office' above a door had been a stark reminder of my reduced circumstances and lowered status.

The counselling course had shown me the power of the mind: that how we deal with stress can affect how we feel. I'd decided that survival lay in viewing this Dickensian scene as spectator, rather than player and in my imagination I'd become an author, soaking up material for my next book – until they'd called me in.

"What income do you have?"

"None." It's getting harder to breathe.

I sit directly in front of the judge. I might as well be in the dock. Oblivious to my surroundings, my eyes plead for clemency. *Will he grant the divorce? Will he allow my son to stay with me?*

"What is your husband paying you?"

"Nothing." My husband still has not arrived.

"Nothing?"

It's reminiscent of hospital consultations: '*What does your husband do? Are you back at work?*'

"No."

I'm a cancer patient without any income. Does this make me an 'unfit mother'?

"What state benefits are you getting?"

"None. I'm told my case has to be decided by an adjudicator because I am doing a part time educational course. It could take months." I can hardly breathe and force the words out. I must appear strong, calm, capable – well-balanced. *Keep eye contact. No tears.*

"When did you last get in touch with them?"

"This morning."

Silence. He consults papers.

"Well they'd better hurry up and do something." He sounds rattled. I don't know if he's annoyed with me, or for me.

When, finally, I escape, I still don't know what decisions will be made. Later I learn my husband's presence had not been required.

Chapter 48

Doors
I barricade the doors, I seal the edge
Nothing to pass through
I banish you

Invasive memories, that twist the knife too much
With tender touch

Relentlessly
Slicking through
Back you seep
Infusing me

They have their own laws, these ghosts
They make their own doors

Three months after moving out of the matrimonial home, I still can't eat normal sized meals, but happily self indulge with chocolate bars and ice-creams, trying to gain weight. The pain of defecation brings daily reminders of past ordeals. Not that I need reminding. Playback still plagues me.

I still have no income. Living frugally is a challenge, but I discover the delights of charity shops. The art course is stimulating and therapeutic. The colour begins to flow back into my life, literally and metaphorically, but by the afternoon, I have to support one hand with the other as I paint. When I carry any weight it exacerbates pain in my neck and back and I have to empty low denomination coinage from my purse before going shopping. My sensitivity to odours, smoke and noise is so heightened and my head and whole body so over-sensitive to pain, someone suggests I could have the condition 'ME' (myalgic encephalomyelitis) but I don't want more labels. (Later, I hear that people who push themselves too hard after serious illness are likely to acquire this condition.) Then a pain clinic consultant tells me that long term, unresolved pain could have left nerves permanently affected.

Festering conflict spirals out of control. It's all my fault. I can't communicate with them. I've closed down. But why did I close down? Self-doubt nags at me. *Only I can heal myself – must fight back harder.* In the car, I turn the music up and tell the ghosts to leave me alone.

But as I stand in a queue one day, someone paying her newspaper account identifies herself by number and for a few moments I'm rooted to the spot. I become similarly transfixed when someone on the radio describes being held hostage and tortured. It's the same if anyone says, 'nearly done' or 'nearly there'.

A consultant has prescribed Naproxen 500mg twice daily, for head, neck and back pain, but these only seem to worsen my symptoms. My stomach burns and it feels as if my nervous system's outer coating has been removed. My new GP is quick to spot cause and effect. "Have you lost your elastic?" he jokes, as my skirt settles on skeletal hips. Instead of examining my back, he digs a finger into my stomach.

"How does this feel . . . and this?"

"Aargh!"

He thinks various anti-inflammatory tablets and pain pills prescribed over the past 2 years have been eroding my stomach and intestines (which accounts for the two sore places I'd described to the oncologist). No-one seems to have considered what effect such drugs might have on someone whose intestines had been blasted by chemo-radiation and who can only manage a minimal diet.

When he asks about my home situation and I tell him that being unable to pay the next month's rent doesn't really help my stress levels, he gives me a note to take to the Department of Social Security (DSS). Within a few hours I'm able to collect a back-payment cheque. My son eats well that night.

DISCUSSION

Why were you so affected when the woman identified herself by number?
She was reduced to a number. I found myself momentarily identifying with tattooed concentration camp victims.

But you didn't have a radiotherapy planning tattoo.
No. I think it was a psychological reaction to being controlled – one among thousands – my hospital number.

What needed to change?
Communication between professionals should mean each has an overview and understanding of a patient's medical history.

There needs to be a designated person in primary and in secondary care, who will take responsibility for ensuring all cancer patients receive financial guidance, according to their *changing* needs.

Patient-held records, as devised by Measham Medical Unit,[46] could ensure patient needs were being addressed.

Chapter 49

My support for an elderly neighbour results in an invitation to become a member of the local Community Health Council (CHC) – known informally as 'The Patients' Watchdog'. Although it has few 'teeth', members have a statutory right of entry into NHS Trusts. Taking part in hospital inspections helps me climb from the lowly position of 'patient', (one who is 'done-to, controlled') to a person of some command, while training, monthly meetings and interaction with local health trusts and authorities educate me into the ways and workings of the NHS. I learn to interpret 'jargonese' and marvel as issues are deflected with spin worthy of any politician.

Patients in the support group always crave more cancer information, so I arrange a nurse speaker from a drugs company. Although the CHC kindly allows me to pin a poster advertising her talk, 'The Side Effects of Cancer Treatments', on their notice-board in the local hospital, an irate surgeon soon rips it down. The hospital social worker who runs the group is called to account and, shaking in her shoes, tells me that patients are not supposed to know there are such things as 'side effects'! Support group members laugh incredulously.

Shortly afterwards she resigns. Despite debilitating levels of ongoing fatigue, I find myself running the group. We put together a library of information, get leaflets printed, write good practice guidelines, a directory of local and national services and send out a monthly newsletter with a circulation of up to ninety. Two of us attend CancerLink's 'Good Practice for Groups' training and the group is one of the first in the country to attend their 'user involvement' training – preparing us to work with health professionals to influence change. But new members still ask us why staff at the local hospital told them there were no local support groups. There seems to be ongoing opposition to independent support groups.

Maggie Jencks' brave story[47] and her project to build a cancer care centre at the Western General Hospital, Edinburgh, inspire me. I attend a 2-day course at Mount Vernon Hospital, Middlesex, on how to set up such a centre, visit several similar centres and collect a file of information on what other areas are providing. Although I cannot get our local hospital interested in providing such a service, the file proves useful in the future and later, the support group achieves recognition.[48]

As secretary of the cancer support group, I receive newsletters from CancerLink and through them learn about Bristol Cancer Help Centre (now 'Penny Brohn Cancer Care').[49] It's hard to contain my excitement when I'm told a week's convalescence will be funded by Social Services. Two months later, I'm on my way south.

In a beautiful Georgian building furnished like a comfortable country home, we soak up the healing and learn to 'let go'. Here, staff have time to care. Here is kindness, warmth, compassion. Here, patients become people again and people in pieces are made whole.

I know nothing of the complementary therapies on offer and admit I have tended to lump them together with alternative medicines as 'quackery', but I try out Shiatsu, a type of massage. The effect of a caring touch is unexpected and overwhelming. Next moment I'm crying as though I will never stop.

My consultation with their lady doctor is different from anything I have ever experienced. She talks to me as an equal. She listens with empathy and understanding, and without seeming rushed. I learn how to access another oncologist, so that I can continue to be followed-up.

Returning home semi-healed, but still suffering playback and conflict, I'm convinced the only way to lay my ghosts is to effect change. There is nothing for it – I will have to beard the lion in his den.

It's good of him to see me, since I'm no longer his patient. I'm shaking with nervousness.

"I think you are one of the good guys, but I need to know for sure." (Still can't control my mouth, you see, counselling course notwithstanding.) "Please would it be possible to tell GPs what to expect when patients are sent home to be ill, at the end of the first four weeks of treatment?"

"I can't tell a GP when to visit!" he protests.

"No, but you can tell them what side-effects might be likely and what help they might need," I reason, gently.

"We can't know. Every patient reacts differently."

But you have a darned good idea!

"Please will you ensure patients are given pre-medication and effective pain relief straight after the implant procedure in theatre, before the connection to radioactivity?"

"There's nothing wrong with the system."

There was for me!

"About the rectal examination . . ." my breathing is so shallow, I can barely speak, "you went on pushing and pushing."

"Yes."

Strange. I had expected a denial. *Why was it done that way? Why didn't you offer me pain relief?* But I cannot say what needs to be said.

"You can't expect to come here and tell me what to do," he says pleasantly, but implacably.

"I'm not trying to tell you what to do, I'm pleading with you – appealing to your humanity," I implore, knowing this is probably my only chance to get things changed. I can't cope with stress and confrontation is bringing me close to tears. All I have is resolve, and it's not enough. But he is obdurate.

How can things improve unless there is acknowledgement that something needs to change? Powerful people have commensurate responsibility. Christmas brings an opportunity to prod. I send him a giant humbug. *(People who feel they have no voice . . .)*

DISCUSSION

Did the reply, 'every patient reacts differently' satisfy you?
No. This phrase is often used to avoid acknowledging the effects of treatment, or to avoid giving patients honest answers.

What did the interview achieve?
Nothing. As it became clear there was no chance of resolution, I became even more stressed and inarticulate. I felt guilty for raising issues when I owed him my life and later actually wrote an apologetic letter, hoping to open his mind to change.

What needed to change?
A team approach to cancer patient care was needed.
  Patients need a key contact within the team as a support.
  Patients need to be able to raise serious issues with their team, rather than with an individual.

Chapter 50

Castle Howard Hussies

Flaunting ladies of the park
Shake off winter's sombre dark
Don magic mists of greenery
Put on ephemeral dreamery
Pirouette the scenery
And dance!

Layered petticoats ruffling high
Shimmering flounces net the sky
Grannies, with arthritic knees
Are chorus girls, all dressed to please
Do an encore, flirt and tease
And dance!

Though painful joints be stiff and set
Make haste, before the spring has met
With summer's dull and dumpy spread
Bold autumn splashes all in red
And winter puts you back to bed –
Now dance!

The divorce has gone through without any problems. Not only has my son not been taken away from me, my daughter has been made redundant and come to live with us. She sleeps on the settee, her legs hanging over the end. And the dogs now live in the garage! Either could mean eviction if the landlady finds out. But it won't be for long because the good news is, after two years, our smallholding has been sold.

When we went back to collect my remaining belongings, we found the dogs were to be put down, so we squashed them into the car among the boxes, and left that place forever. Cardboard boxes and charity shop blankets insulate them against the night cold. We just hope they don't bark.

I have 6 months to find a new home, after which the DSS starts taking a proportion of my capital. The race is on. Town or country? I still find it difficult to make decisions and am grateful for my daughter's assistance. Never one for the easy road, I buy a country cottage with 'potential' and in May 1994, four years after the end of treatment, we move to our new home. The approach road is lined with magnificent trees, for all-the-world like crinolined ladies and the inspiration for my first non-cancer 'pome', 'Castle Howard Hussies'. We survive winter without central heating, living in a virtual building site during extensive renovations, but my designer daughter decorates the house on a shoe-string budget and in spring we have roses round the door.

The new GP is very pleasant and I'm hopeful of building up a rapport, but when I try to tell him about the playback of traumatic events I'm still experiencing he cuts me short with, "So *you* say!"

Figment

A Thing apart am I
A happening, touched with a Romany need
Restless I flee, forever seeking

Lone traveller, moonkissed am I
Inconstant changeling, firefly
I flit between the stars
You hear me soughing as an autumn breeze
And keening is my cry

A passing thought am I, half seen
A haunting, part-glimpsed from the corner of an eye
Wraithlike, spiriting the land
Then with the merest flicker of a lash
Evaporating to a dream

Torn fragment of cloud am I
No salt upon my tail
I ride the crests, wave borne.
Knowing no rest, I conquer sleep
Just as the Deep

What cage could hold the echo of a memory?
Free must I fly
If tethered but a single day, I fret and die

I'm now a degree student, a member of the Community Health Council and heavily involved in voluntary work. Life should be back on track, but it's not. A balance between constipation from pain pills and the effects of Lactulose syrup is hard to achieve, while daily pain and fatigue ensure ongoing isolation. This is no ordinary tiredness. I have no stamina and after the slightest exertion I feel ill and long to lie down. All my joints ache. The oncologist had said radiotherapy would go on working for years and from what I have learned I've guessed that the massive amount I had is the reason further treatments are not an option. Being super sensitive to cold, cigarette smoke, exhaust fumes and noise is now 'normal' to me. I have urinary and faecal urgency. There is ongoing pain.

Cancer charities' patient information does not prepare me for these problems. It does not supply the individual detail most patients seek and even seems to ape medical paternalism with its 'protective' omissions and positive generalisations. There is no booklet on anal cancer. I do not realise that booklets on gynaecological cancers contain information that is likely to apply to me (such as side effects of pelvic radiotherapy). It grieves me to read that hair loss is supposedly 'temporary', when mine has not grown back. Loss of my pubic hair is having more effect on me than I would have imagined. I feel a freak. Successive GPs have told me they don't know anything about the side effects of cancer treatments. (Later, when discussing lymphoedema with my new oncologist after breast

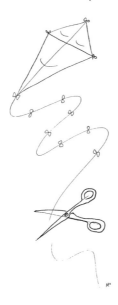

Figure 50.1 Figment.

cancer treatment, I mention that three-quarters of my body has been 'radiotherapied', but even she does not seem to be aware of what treatments I have had and says 'Surely not that much'. The earlier treatment had become more targeted by then. I feel no-one has an understanding of my difficulties.)

It's a struggle to keep the house clean and there's no spare energy for socialising. Just as well, with my uncertain future I feel it wouldn't be fair to make close friends or have a personal relationship. I'm just a liability. In college, I look on enviously as a group of students regularly get together for a chat and biscuits at coffee time. Only after coverage in the local newspaper (as spokesperson for the support group) does the class realise I've had cancer and one of those envied offers me a chocolate biscuit. "I'm so sorry", he says. "We didn't know." After that, I'm invited to join them each day. Cancer has gained me entry to the club!

Ghosts still batter at my head: trauma playback as vivid as original experiences; too many unanswered questions; hurt conflicting with indebtedness. I'm envious when I hear of trauma victims being offered counselling.

When an endoscopic investigation, prompted by stomach pain, causes no discomfort thanks to a throat spray and sedation, I can only wonder why I was not offered similar relief for the rectal examination. The inconsistency is hard to take.

Some people who learn my cancer treatment had not included surgery exclaim, "Weren't you lucky!" Yes, I was lucky. I am lucky. I just wish I could feel lucky!

I write to the BMA Medical Ethics Committee regarding consent. They reply, 'the basic premise is that treatment is undertaken as a result of patients being actively involved in deciding what is to be done to them'. Then why doesn't this happen?

The experiences of people within the support group make me realise how much is wrong with cancer services, although none of those who had operations had significant pain. The same issues are raised repeatedly: communication, information and consent; diagnostic and treatment delays; ambulance transport; lack of support and pain relief; inadequate nursing care and monitoring of chemotherapy patients. Patient after patient asks 'Why do we have to fight for information? It's hard enough having cancer, without having to deal with this on top." The stories of 'too-late diagnoses' are so common, I come to expect them. Cancer seems last on the list of possibilities. People are dying unnecessarily, but no-one is speaking out. Patients don't complain because they feel vulnerable and they can't deal with extra stress; bereaved relatives are too debilitated by grief; hospital and hospice staff, who must be aware of these silent undercurrents, seem unable to make public what they hear. The issues get buried along with the patients.

I wonder at what point doctors become de-humanized and whether it is inevitable.[50] What is the cause: training, culture, systems, pressures; the 'enthusiasm for business and science'? It is salutary when a doctor asks such questions and patently admits doctors are *not* humane to patients.[51]

How can I get on with my life while people continue to suffer unnecessarily? How can I speak out when I can't talk about things without crying; when I might frighten other patients into refusing treatment?

Chapter 51

Tomorrow People
Tipped into battle, culled
Unwilling conscripts in a never-ending war
For this is the Forgotten Zone
No easy track, with serpents heads in view
To slide you back

But veterans among the chosen few
Now set upon a different plane
Might keep in mind the raw recruits to follow

Who else is there to keep the score
For the Tomorrow People
And how many more?

1994 marks a turning point. The government wants to give patients a voice and I'm invited to a conference on the theme of 'Patient Empowerment'. When we divide into workshops, I seize the opportunity to fill a dreaded flip chart and, finally empowered to speak out, expound on general cancer issues in front of the whole group (I'm getting braver!). In the plenary session, my comment about GP 'too-late' referrals is the only item of feedback to get spontaneous applause. Inadvertently I have become a patient advocate and campaigner. I write a paper for the CHC on the cancer issues, including a call for a cancer help centre at the hospital, and send it to the local Health Authority, local health trusts and other statutory organisations. The Medical Director of one hospital says he will share it with consultants, but then there is silence.

Although soon commuted to 'patient partnership', the NHS patient empowerment initiative marks the dawning of an unofficial patient 'movement' that is to prompt a massive culture-change in healthcare. Increasing numbers of patients and patient representatives begin to speak out. At first their voices are mere raindrops in a pond, but each causes ripples. The experiences of one member of our group inspire her to write a novel.[52]

It's still difficult to articulate my experiences. Writing articles gradually helps to sort out the tangles, and getting them published in patient magazines gives me a voice.[53,54] Caring passionately gives me the courage to give presentations but mostly I'm preaching to the converted, when I need to be raising awareness among 'Them'.

The local press is not slow to realise I am willing to speak out on behalf of the support group and often asks me to comment on topical cancer issues. Interested only in contention, they never print positive remarks I make about local health services, still, 'any publicity is good publicity' and I'm happy to put my head on the block if it means the group gets free promotion, although the labels 'cancer sufferer' and worse, 'cancer victim', sit uneasily. I live,

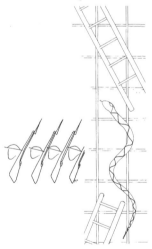

Figure 51.1 Tomorrow people.

breathe and dream cancer and to my long-suffering friends and family, became without question, a cancer bore.

People assume I'm 'putting something back' and smile in admiration. But I don't see myself as altruistic. I don't have a choice. I'm driven. Life has become a quest for truth; a mystery to be solved; a need for change.

Rush hour
Boot-licking city-slickers
Shoulder-snitching money-grubbers
Thigh rubbers, waist huggers
Legs locked, feet squashed
Shoes squeak, protestingly
Plasticised people with microchip matter
Returning on cue to homogenised homes
'Civilised society', melded in the melting pot
Riding the Production Line.
The staleness in your eyes belies your affluence

Blank faces, vacant spaces
Cloned drones with yellowed skin
Where is your hope, your enterprise, endeavour?
How could you begin to gauge the measure
Of my ascetic pleasure?

One thing leads to another. Voluntary involvement at national level as a Trustee Director of CancerLink and on the Advisory Council of the National Cancer Alliance (professionals and patients trying to improve cancer services) is valuable experience and boosts my confidence. My knowledge of cancer increases, as does my medical vocabulary. Certain words resonate and are squirreled away: 'palliative care'; 'iatrogenic pain' (pain caused unintentionally by a doctor).

Travelling to London makes me acutely aware of my impoverished state, yet I take pride in managing to live at subsistence level and find fulfilment in what I am doing. Crammed into the Tube in my charity shop clothes, I feel richer than my pale-faced commuter companions.

Peace of mind remains elusive. I don't brood about things: *they* invade *me*. Although totally indebted to staff who saved my life, I still need to know why certain things happened and crave acknowledgement of what was wrong.

In order to find out what is good practice regarding follow up examinations and pain relief for implants, I write to several consultants in other areas. It's incredibly nerve-wracking to confront the gods. I'm 'only a patient', still a stick insect suffering daily pain and debility. I can't even touch on the issue of lack of consent, but reason if pain relief were to be offered, at least patients would have to be told an examination was imminent.

Most do not reply and one ticks me off for referring to doctors 'furthering their education'. But two in particular confirm the need for pain relief when connecting implants and inscribe their names on my brain for the openness of their responses and the humanity of their practice. "If examination were necessary *at that time*," writes one, with regard to the rectal examination, "the only recourse would be general anaesthetic."

The pain and shock of the rectal examination has affected me more than the pain of the implant connection, so this acknowledgement of the need for change is a great comfort, but I need action. A nurse suggests asking the hospital if what happened to me is still happening. I write in all innocence, expecting my letter to be taken at face value. The reply ignores my questions and, because they are aware of my work with the support group, suggests I should not be counselling other patients if I have unresolved issues.

When I learn of the Declaration of Patients' Rights in Europe, I write to the World Health Organization (WHO). Their reply makes me want to weep. "It is exactly because of the kind of experiences that you are describing in your letter why WHO has taken the initiative to promote the adoption of patients' rights legislation . . ." they write. "We will try to do all we can in order that patients in Europe would not be exposed to the kind of experience you have had to go through." This touches on acknowledgement of what I went through, but their words are only aspirational.

A Medical Director from another hospital expresses surprise that doctors coming from abroad to learn a technique took an active part in my care, as only those registered with the General Medical Council are allowed to treat patients. In order to check this out, I ask for the name of the doctor who connected the implants, but the hospital claims the handwriting is illegible. I ask for the names of all four foreign doctors who had come to learn the technique. Many months later they reply that their computer system has changed and none of this information is available.

I still feel wrapped in barbed wire. It's extremely difficult to write to the hospital again, repeating my original questions (challenging those who have saved my life) but, in an extraordinary response, a senior nurse manager makes the hundred miles round trip to my new home.

It's very hard to tell her about my experiences. I have to leave the room to compose myself first and as I talk it's a continuous struggle to fight back tears. She seems shocked by what she hears. I've been living with it for over four years. Later I realise we've talked through the lunch hour and I've never even offered her a second cup of coffee.

She asks if I want to make a formal complaint, but I'm adamant I don't want to make trouble for anyone, I just need to know these things are not still happening. No-one can tell me why the rectal examination was done at that time (let alone in that manner) rather than later, but a senior hospital manager says they will try to implement change informally. Meanwhile, relaxation tapes and head-sets are freed from the cupboard, 'Friends of the Hospital' buy a selection of combs and mirrors to offer patients who are admitted as emergencies and a new bench is installed half-way up the 'mountain', to break the journey from car park to hospital entrance. They congratulate me on my achievements and seem to think I should be satisfied with these minor improvements.

The first article submitted to a medical journal is painfully extruded through tears in 1996.[33]

"You'd better not be ill again!" warns my son, anticipating possible reprisals.

"You don't understand," I tell him. I feel so scarred, there's nothing worse they can do to me.

Shredded, but triumphant, I sit back and wait for the flak. Sure enough, the cry of 'foul!' soon blots the letters page with a protest against this 'invasion' and a call to hear from happy and satisfied patients for a change.

Criticism must be hard to accept in a caring profession. I stand guilty as charged. But if there is to be any mutual understanding, we need to talk to each other – invade each others' safe spaces. How can there be any progress if we hide in our own back yards?

'Them' and 'Us' need to become 'We'.

One consultant contacts me to say, after reading my story she is changing her practice and will try to influence that of her colleagues. One is a start.

A year after the nurse's home visit, mindful of the BMA response, I write to see if they have had any success in getting things changed informally. She replies, 'informed consent is still a difficult issue at this hospital'. The manager tells me that is the oncologist's preferred way of working. I am gutted. But my letter sets a formal complaint process in motion. It's the very thing I've been trying to avoid, but how else can I have peace of mind? From wanting to be their 'best ever patient', I'm about to become a pariah.

DISCUSSION

How did you feel when you found a consultant who advocated the use of general anaesthetic for the rectal examination?
I felt vindicated. His compassion held out a hand to me.

They said you should not have been counselling other patients when you had unresolved issues?
In a general sense, they were right, although it was inappropriate to point this out in their reply. Had counselling been provided by the NHS, I would not have had to do it. Other cancer patients did not share my most traumatic experiences and I could enable them to resolve their issues. One Sunday, for example, 5 adult brothers and sisters came to my house. Another brother, who lived in Canada, was dying from cancer, but they did not speak about this to him, or to each other. The meeting gave them the opportunity to share their thoughts and fears for the first time and to decide what action to take.

What needed to change?
Staff and patients could benefit from open, blame-free reporting and learning systems, such as that used in the aircraft industry to minimise risk, and from professional counselling services.

Chapter 52

The emotional and psychological effect of complaining about those who have saved my life becomes as damaging as the systems I'm trying to improve. Half of me hates myself. I feel like a traitor, but this is probably my last chance to protect future patients and gain peace of mind. I'm still a physical and emotional wreck, yet, just as with the divorce proceedings, I have to appear strong and credible if I'm to have a chance of success.

In order to get at the truth, I obtain copies of my medical records, which reveal some surprising anomalies. There is a tick beside 'transport required', although transport had not been offered. I note I'd had '40.00 Gy in 20 fractions to lower pelvis and groins' – although on another page it says, correctly, 'to the whole pelvis'. While this is a minor blip, more startling is that my diagnosis had been 'squamous carcinoma', yet 'basaloid' is written in my notes.

I find details of my treatment, ('Mitomycin C and 5FU according to the protocol; 20.00 Gy in 10 fractions to the left groin; iridium wire implantation . . . 25.00 Gy to the 85% isodose') which could have given me a knowledge base if I'd had them at the beginning. At least now I know the name of the 'expensive' wire – all 4 syllables!

'According to the protocol' intrigues me. Which protocol? 'According to the clinical trial protocol', I'm told. This really surprises me because, shortly after treatment had ended, I'd chanced upon an article about an anal cancer clinical trial at my radiotherapy centre, stating that a 'fourteenth patient' with this 'uncommon neoplasm' had been recently been recruited to the study, which the Gastrointestinal Tumour Group was 'very keen' to support.[55] I'd wondered what a clinical trial was, whether I had been recruited and why no-one had told me about it.

The hospital now says I was definitely not recruited to the trial because I had not met the 'very precise criteria', but I discover even patients with distant metastases had been included.[56] Checking my medical records against recruitment criteria, I find all my test results had been normal (HB 13.4, WBC 7.2, platelets 250) and my records even state I was 'healthy apart from cancer'. I'd had no 'previous treatment for anal cancer' or 'radiotherapy to the pelvis' and no 'history of cancer in other sites'. In fact, I seem to have met all criteria admirably.

There's more. I learn that the simultaneous treatment I'd had is called Combined Modality Therapy (CMT), which is more aggressive than giving chemotherapy and radiotherapy separately (which perhaps accounts for the consultant's assumed nonchalance when I began both treatments). In fact, I read there had been 6 deaths attributed to this chemotherapy in the United Kingdom Co-ordinating Committee on Cancer Research (UKCCCR) trial and there were some who reasoned that patients with early tumours (like mine) have very good results after radiotherapy alone.[9] In the radiotherapy alone arm there were two deaths caused by radiotherapy and two as a consequence of salvage surgery.[57]

I realise that treatment can vary according to clinical preference and can be pioneering, and therefore aggressive (apparently clinicians do not like clinical trial treatments to be referred to as 'experimental') although patients are not told about this.

Protocol modifications[58] written a year before my treatment, hold more surprises. I certainly did not have 'prophylactic antibiotics' (recommended for all patients in the combined modality arm of the trial). Whether or not I was in the trial, the date of the modifications indicates serious side effects of this treatment had been known about before I was sent home to be 'a bit ill'.

Feedback from the parallel quality of life study[59] stated 'Clinicians undoubtedly under-reported morbidity in the trial; for example the majority of patients had a brisk skin reaction which, although expected, should have been noted as morbidity'. 'Brisk' does not adequately describe the effects on me.

It's chilling. But it's absolutely paralysing to read that, after the initial 4-week treatment, the protocol allowed a 6–8 week gap before examination and assessment to allow the area to heal.

DISCUSSION

How did you feel when you discovered combination treatments were more aggressive than single treatments?
Patronised. I wished they could have talked to me about this.

How did you feel when you read that the rectal examination could have been done up to 8 weeks after the end of treatment?
Shocked and worthless.

What needed to change?
If the seriousness of my situation and potential side effects of treatment had been acknowledged, my needs might have been met, my suffering minimised.

A team approach and shared decision-making might have brought humanity into my care.

Chapter 53

Paternalism, the fight for information and the process of being processed (and devalued *as a matter of routine*) have caused far more stress than the cancer itself. Even close friends don't understand why the need to improve cancer services has become such an obsession, or why I seem so detached, even taciturn. I have a great need for the medical profession to understand. 'We need to speak to each other' repeats and repeats in my mind.

Hoping to raise awareness among a larger group of health professionals, I submit an article to the prestigious *British Medical Journal* (*BMJ*) and, incredibly, it's accepted.[34] This is indeed a time of change.

The depth of understanding shown by doctors' commentaries,[60,61] has a powerful healing impact on me. I read their words over and over again, soaking up solace from their acknowledgement of my suffering. Interestingly, the letters of response show views from either end of the spectrum: one takes understanding to an even higher level[62] while another eminently illustrates to the medical profession at large why change is needed.[63]

The supportive doctors join the one who had recommended the use of general anaesthetic for the rectal examination in a 'virtual' treasure chest collection of patient-centred doctors in my mind. I realise I am still searching for compassion.

Membership of the CHC over 8 years keeps me updated on NHS changes, and gives me hope of improving health services locally. Meanwhile patients' stories continue to flood in, compelling me to campaign.

Through the CHC, and in the name of the support group, I lobby the local District Hospital to provide a counselling service for cancer patients. This meets with little response, although a year later their in-house magazine proudly advertises a new counselling service for staff.[64]

However, I am invited to join the joint NHS Trust/CHC Art in Hospital group and the Local Research Ethics Committee. As speaker and 'simulated patient' in medical education elsewhere, I'm privileged to see diagnostic and communication skills blossom. When invited to speak at a 2-day conference on communication issues in cancer care, I am amazed when the Chairman, a palliative care consultant, actually encourages me to speak out about the unnecessary pain I endured and incidents that still plague me.

With the aid of the CHC I'm able to get the Cancer Centre's general information booklet changed to reflect the active role that doctors learning new techniques may play in patients' care. (Sadly, later, during my three-week stay for radiotherapy for breast cancer in 1997, no patients on my ward were given the booklets. When I tackled the male nurse about this, he said, "If we told patients all their rights, there would be lots of things we wouldn't be able to do to them.")

Health professionals, perhaps feeling bruised by the rising tide of patient advocacy, raise frequent reminders that they can get cancer too. But the doctor-turned-patient can never suffer the vulnerability, powerlessness and hurt of the ingenuous patient, totally ignorant of medical cultures and systems. Also, patients often do not know what the hospital policies are, so are powerless for that reason,[65] whereas doctor-patients can use their knowledge of policies and guidelines to circumvent them or gain advantage.

Patient-centred doctors' articles that reflect humility as they admit to shortcomings,[20] have glued a few cracks in this Humpty-Dumpty. And how good it is to learn that some doctors recognise the emotional and psychological problems associated with illness and call for patient testimonies to be heard and acted upon.[66]

Improvements in cancer services and more targeted, less aggressive treatments mean I can speak out without frightening new patients. At the annual National Conference of Cancer Self Groups, hundreds of patients echo the need for more information, better communication, pain relief and support, and share their views with health professionals. Cancer charities join up and became more proactive, patients' voices begin to be heard at the highest level, their views endorsed by patient-centred clinicians. 'Mitzi Mouse' finds herself giving presentations nationally and even internationally.

One day, the local District Hospital Chief Executive surprises me by declaring, "When I retire, I shall be a campaigner. I shall campaign on behalf of old people, because I shall be one!" It seems one of 'Them' actually respects what I am trying to do.

DISCUSSION

Do you think your expectations were too high?
Was it too much to expect honesty? In retrospect I could see my perceptions had become so twisted by insecurity, I was over-analytical and over-critical about the smallest detail. But what had caused this?

'There is no certainty; there is only adventure. Even stars explode.'

Roberto Assagioli

PART III

Chapter 54 ▬

"How on earth did your GP manage to take a smear? I can't even see your cervix."

It's 8 years since the anal cancer diagnosis, but only a year since my second major challenge: unrelated breast cancer. The drug 'Tamoxifen' has caused vaginal bleeding and a different consultant is examining me prior to checking my uterus for endometrial cancer (a side effect of the drug) under general anaesthetic.

This is how I learn the 'nasty surprises' have not quite finished with me and radiation damage has caused vaginal adhesions. (I'd never heard of 'adhesions'.) So parts of the body really can stick together – parts I had not even realised could be at risk. When I had mentioned urinary problems to my GP, she'd said a prolonged stream became common as women aged and quoted a patient's husband as saying, 'My wife no longer pees like a horse'. *'Ha! Ha!'* Now I learn my bladder opening (urethra) and surrounding tissue is inflamed and my uterus is fused and pulled sideways so the cervix is out of sight.

Only now do they provide vaginal dilators that can prevent adhesions and other radiotherapy side effects. Why wasn't I given these at the time? Forming close relationships after cancer can be difficult enough, without such problems adding to isolation. *Were they in denial about this, too?[67] Did these things not matter, not figure in their quality of life assessments? Was life after fifty (or sixty, seventy . . .) presumed to be devoid of sex? Would it be the same if their own lives were affected?* My GP's remark, 'adhesions are very common' holds no comfort.

(A week beforehand, I had discovered from a friend that a dilatation and curettage procedure (D&C or 'scrape') was usually done whenever they 'took a look' at the uterus under general anaesthetic and the consultant confirms this. I tell her I would appreciate being told in advance of anything they plan to do and she says it is 'just routine'. *But I need to know the routine!* They say they will also take a look to check for radiation damage in my backside at the same time, but I am in agony on the loo the next day and later read in my notes that they had taken 4 tissue samples from my anal canal.)

Adhesions are not the only surprise. Twelve years after treatment, and just as the twenty-first century begins to hold promise, truncal (abdominal) lymphoedema (a break-down of the body's lymphatic system) makes its presence felt, along with a diagnosis of 'venous insufficiency' in my legs. Both my GP and oncologist readily admit they know little about lymphoedema which I discover is a common, if unacknowledged problem.[68]

Slight swelling in the suprapubic area shortly after the end of treatment had been dismissed with, '*should* be temporary'. As my user involvement work had increased, journeys to London had become more frequent – too many days spent sitting on trains and in meetings. Importantly, no-one had mentioned lengthy sitting and immobility would be contra-indicated after double doses of radiation to lymph nodes in the groin.

I contact the Lymphoedema Support Network (LSN), a wonderful organisation run from St Luke's Crypt, Sydney Street, London SW3 6NH, which supports patients and tries to raise awareness and improve lymphoedema services. From a journal[69] they supply, I learn about a collaborative initiative, The Lymphoedema Framework Project, which 'aims to provide evidence that lymphoedema is a major problem, under-resourced, needing specific national guidance, so that ultimately all patients receive appropriate assessment and treatment'. Although the journal indicates the need for early intervention, I cannot access treatment or a lymphoedema specialist. I learn that the hospice-run clinic receives a pot of money from the Primary Care Trust (PCT) but none is ring-fenced for lymphoedema.

As my body continues to swell, I feel as if I am fighting for my life because, without quality, there *is* no life. Sitting as the (unpaid) lay representative on a Department of Health pathology modernisation group, yet abandoned to the horrors and potential complications of this progressive condition, becomes an increasingly surreal experience. A precious year is lost, battling, before I am allowed a 'one-off' course of Manual Lymphatic Drainage (MLD) treatment. Although it is successful (3 litres of fluid lost) I cannot routinely access further treatment.

DISCUSSION

How did you feel when you realised they were about to do a D & C without telling you, and also that they had taken biopsies after saying they would just take a look?
I was dreadfully disappointed. This was 8 years after my previous experiences of paternalism and I had read so much guidance setting out patient-centred care, yet it seemed to be a paper exercise. I was still trying to trust them.

How did you feel when late radiation effects appeared?
My life had been saved, so I do not wish to appear ungrateful. It is no use weeping for what might have been, but the adhesions could have been prevented and information about lymphoedema might have helped to prevent it developing. At least the effects in my vagina were an indication of what I had suffered in the more targeted area of the anal canal.

What needed to change?
Clinicians should be explicit about their intentions and obtain patient consent well in advance of any action.

Prior to commencing pelvic radiotherapy treatment, all patients should receive information about acute and late effects of radiation on vaginal tissue and this should be recorded within the consent process.

Patients should be supplied with a pack of vaginal dilators and vaginal dilation should be viewed as an integral aspect of post treatment supportive care and rehabilitation (and also used during treatment).[70]

Undergraduate and post-graduate medical education should include raised awareness and training about lymphoedema.

Lymphoedema patients should have equal access to treatment, whatever part of their body is affected.

Lymphoedema services should not have to compete with palliative care services for finance.

Network-wide surveys should be undertaken to establish the real extent of lymphoedema in the community as well as in hospitals.

Service capacity should improve to match patient need according to national guidelines,[71] which should be explicit.

Chapter 55

Dharma
I have seen the garden
I have the key
I can swing the heavy door and know the mystery

There's a magic waiting
Hidden from your eyes
A squandering of daydreams; a harvesting of sighs

If you want the secret
Walk in the dew
Step among the frosted fields and see life anew

See dandelion miracles
Clocks of fairy time
Diamond crusted are their works, jewelled with the rime

See spiders gently bouncing
Trampolines of pearls
Necklacing the garden as the day unfurls

Then you'll know the secret
You can turn the key
Then you'll know awakening
You will be free

The radiotherapy centre eventually apologised for the unnecessary pain I had suffered during the implant connection, although I did not want a meaningless, corporate apology. I simply wanted change. They told me that subsequent anal cancer patients who had iridium implants were given pre-medication and were fitted with patient controlled anaesthesia (pca) machines before theatre as well as receiving a pain-relieving spinal boost. This was acknowledgement of the level of pain I suffered. Patients who received pelvic radiation were also told about side effects and given vaginal dilators to prevent adhesions, vaginal shrinkage etc.

They kindly allowed me to see all the scan slides and explained them to me. It turned out cancer had not spread to my bones and only one side of my pelvis had been affected. The two white blobs I'd seen had been my hip bones!

During an independent review of my treatment, I asked two doctors about my extreme susceptibility to cold, but was told they did not know what effect cancer treatments had on 'humeral substances'. When I asked whether damage from the protracted implant connection could be responsible for the pain I still suffered and what future effects it might have, there was the familiar hesitancy. Then one doctor said it was not likely to make much difference – 'considering the amount of radiotherapy you've had'. Alarm bells were ringing again. I asked them straight out if I would need a colostomy at some future point. They said they did not know. But they were squirming.

I had to turn the question around and ask whether someone who had the same cancer and treatment as me would be likely to need a colostomy in the future.[72] It was incredibly difficult. They followed the usual pattern of looking at each other, then at the floor – but they did not speak. At the end of a particularly gruelling day (the stressful culmination of years of trying to effect change on certain issues) I had to summon every ounce of assertiveness and plead, "Please! I really need to know!"

Even then they could not give a straight answer. "Well," said one, "we always say . . . better to have loved and lost . . ." and then fell silent.

At this juncture, I was close to losing it!

"Seventy to seventy-five percent of people will need a colostomy at some point," he concluded, "Yes."

At last! So it was a colostomy after all – if I didn't die first. Were they saying it was to be expected because they were afraid I would sue? Surely extra tearing and scar tissue would cause loss of normal function earlier than usual? How many more nasty surprises had they got up their sleeves?

Of the rectal examination, their report stated that I had been told what was about to happen and why and that there was 'no protestation made'. (The report also described my staging as 'T2 N2 MO'; the implants' duration as seventy-two hours, instead of sixty; and spoke of separate treatment to right, instead of left, inguinal nodes.)

Some issues are too big; some people too powerful. I had to hope that simply raising the issue might have brought changes – perhaps not admitted to.

DISCUSSION

What did it feel like to learn you would probably need a colostomy at some point?
It was humiliating to think that this information had been withheld from me – as devastating as the news itself. Had I known earlier, I might have ordered my life differently (worn a bikini at every opportunity!) and my appreciation of still being able to do certain things would have been so much greater. Nothing could recapture that.

How did you feel when they procrastinated?
Extremely stressed.

What needed to change?
An immediate explanation of the scan pictures could have prevented years of misunderstandings.
  Patients' questions need to be answered directly and openly.
  Doctors need to be honest with themselves, as well as with patients.

Chapter 56

In 1993, the General Medical Council recommended that communication skills training should be included in the general undergraduate curriculum,[73] although it took years before this became a formal requirement. Most bad news was broken by surgeons and few received formal postgraduate training in this area.[4] However, there was recognition of the need for dialogue with patients, for health professionals to tackle emotive issues[74] and for those involved in cancer care to have good communication skills. Some communication courses were placing importance on helping health professionals acknowledge and deal with their own emotions.[75] Research showed communication skills training for senior oncologists resulted in positive shifts in their attitudes towards patients' psychosocial needs, as well as improved confidence ratings.[76]

Good practice in breaking bad news was spreading: in 1997, following investigations in a breast clinic 'one-stop-shop' (set up after successful lobbying) the specialist breast surgeon prepared me with an opening sentence, "I'm afraid things are not quite as clear-cut as we'd hoped," and went on to explain why my breast lump was almost certainly cancer. That first sentence was so important. It alerted me that, despite my GP's reassurances and the consequent 5 month delay in referral, there was indeed a problem. And it gently allowed me to acknowledge that cancer was the most likely probability.

Calls for a cancer help and information centre at the local district hospital were eventually answered and my file of information about various established centres was used in planning. The support group donated almost £500, raised from sales of home-made items. (It later received official recognition of its services in the form of an award from The All Party Parliamentary Group on Breast Cancer and an £8,000.00 grant from the local Health Authority.)

The General Medical Council told doctors they must listen to patients[29] and that meant taking their views on board. In 1995, The Calman-Hine Report[77] highlighted the need for major changes to cancer services and began a process of development in secondary care and palliative services. Patients' insight, knowledge and involvement in health services were being recognised as 'a powerful and under-utilised force in helping professionals manage change'.[78]

By the end of the nineteen-nineties, although paternalism was recognised as being 'endemic in the NHS . . . yet out of step with society',[79] power would not be relinquished easily, as critics of 'benevolent arrogance' were likely to discover.[80,81]

However, in 2000, the NHS Plan[82] and the NHS Cancer Plan[83] brought more changes, driving forwards the evolution of consumer advocacy and reiterating the call for all cancer treatment in England to be based on Multidisciplinary Team (MDT) working.

The establishment of Cancer Networks with their service user groups and partnership working meant cancer patients at last had a valid voice and could attempt to change the culture and power balance in what had formerly been 'foreign territory'. The ripples on the pond began to join up. Understandably, in the early days there was some tokenism, which still lingers in NHS 'backwaters' where the concept of genuine user involvement has yet to be understood (incredibly, even today, some partnership groups are still chaired by health professionals and patients are allowed to attend the first day of a conference, but not the second). But patients and professionals were communicating with one another and learning the benefits of working together.[84]

It was comforting to find acknowledgement that palliative care could be needed early in cancer treatment: 'It is the right of every person with a life-threatening illness to receive appropriate palliative care wherever they are and at whatever stage of their illness'.[85] In 2004, guidance was published which aimed to ensure that the needs of cancer patients and their families and carers were addressed at all stages of the disease.[71]

Clinicians were realising that most patients wanted more information[86] and antiquated, 'not in front of the children' attitudes, were being replaced by openness, in recognition of twenty-first century patients' needs. It was very satisfying to know that the cancer issues I had raised with statutory bodies so long ago were now being addressed.

In 2006, the General Medical Council issued new supplementary guidance, 'Maintaining Boundaries',[87] which supplied more detail on how to comply with the principles in their guidance, 'Good Medical Practice', including what doctors must do and what they must tell patients before carrying out intimate examinations.

My cancer poems were dusted down and used in medical journals, medical education, to inform the planning team designing a new cancer centre and as the basis for a therapeutic writing workshop. A friend felt inspired to put some to music and we compiled a 'music and poetry-readings' CD to raise money for charity (Macmillan Cancer Support and the Lymphoedema Support Network).

When a Cancer Network Director and Lead Clinician asked me to contribute to his book, *Modernising Cancer Services*, it felt as if we had reached a milestone.[72] Pariah no more?

Chapter 57

The Calman-Hine Report[77] had made no specific recommendations for primary care, which left patients reliant on local initiatives, but guidance in 2004[88] brought together the experience of leaders in the field, and, encouragingly, the late and long term side effects of cancer treatment were at last being acknowledged. In 2006, Macmillan Cancer Support's report *Yesterday's Women*,[89] aimed to stimulate discussion about chronic survivorship conditions in general and the late effects of radiation treatment in particular. Among the six areas they highlighted for attention was the need to improve communication between primary and secondary care and for a national register of the consequences of cancer treatment.

However, a year later, official patient radiotherapy information[90] still did not acknowledge that serious side effects could occur many years after treatment, only that 'some begin during treatment and some could appear weeks or even months afterwards'. Surprisingly, it mentioned that radiotherapy could cause anaemia, which could even necessitate a blood transfusion. This might have accounted for my breathlessness and exhaustion. I wondered why I had not had the 'regular blood tests during treatment'.

At the parliamentary launch of the Macmillan report, I was lucky enough to meet a rather special GP, Dr Pawan Randev, with whom I had been in correspondence years before. (I had been overcome with admiration when I read of the innovative work of doctors, Pawan Randev and Orest Mulka from the Measham Medical Unit,[91] who, in 1997, had begun a project to apply accreditation principles to primary care and devised their own patient-held record. The information pack they kindly sent made me wonder why this level of care should be exceptional, rather than usual – and why it was not compulsory for all GP practices.)

It was at this meeting that Dr Randev made the suggestion that GPs should receive follow-up letters at each phase of cancer treatment (this could have ensured GP support and prevented my suffering mid-way through treatment – *see* Chapter 23). Once active treatment was complete, an overall summary would allow linkage and identification of the key letter in a time limited consultation and also would set the clinical agenda regarding the cancer for years so that it might be possible to link up new signs and symptoms to related treatments.

He later mentioned another important patient safety issue that he had been working on: that drugs initiated, dispensed and monitored by secondary or tertiary care should be added to the GP prescribing screen by GPs. They would then always be prompted about side effects and possible interactions with medication. This area is a significant, unrecognised source of potential prescribing errors which has particular relevance to primary care clinical trials of medication. An editorial in *Prescriber*[92] describes how a solution has been achieved in his own practice (while awaiting the integrated patient record). A positive response from the National Patient Safety Agency gives hope that these ideas will be taken forwards.[93] My patient and professional colleagues in cancer user groups certainly hope so, and would like see both these, and the recommendations in Macmillan's report,[89] embedded in national guidance. (Dr Randev can be contacted by email at: pawan.randev@nhs.net or telephone.)[91]

Dr Randev joined other gems in my 'virtual' treasure chest, such as the GP I met who encourages his patients to write their own referral letter, which he sends along with his own. He finds additional information emerges when patients have time to recall symptoms at home.

In patients' eyes, these are the 'great' men of medicine – the doctors whom patients will remember with admiration, awe and even affection.

Chapter 58

Self heal
I built defences strong and tall
A wall within
To stop Barbarians pouring through
Overpowering, devouring
Invading everything

I fought until, with weapons spent, I woke
Spell broken
Barricade of glass, bright shards
And saw the forces gathered like a sea
Were mine
My loyal army, battling to help me win
The sole invader of my mind was me

During treatment, I had not realised there was such a thing as a psychological side to having cancer. Later, I wondered what percentage of patients' psychological problems were attributable to cancer *care* (paternalism, lack of, and conflicting information), rather than cancer itself, and if anyone had dared to research this. When I came across deep understanding of the devastating effects of medical deceit it healed another crack.[94]

The counselling course had shown me how to overcome stress, but still could not eradicate the replay. Only by improving services could my ghosts be laid to rest. Fortunately, the aftermath of cancer had given me the freedom to choose what to do with my life. No longer defined by my lowest point, I'd shed my 'cancer patient' skin and became 'patient advocate, medical writer and artist'. But my immersion in medical matters, and cancer in particular, had not been comfortable for others and was perhaps regarded as an eccentricity. Concerned friends had urged me to 'get on with my life'. "You can't change the world, Mitzi!" they'd said. Some things one cannot change. Sometimes change happens without acknowledgement of influencing forces. Does it matter, as long as improvements are made?

Medical schools would seem to hold the key to bringing humanity into cancer care, yet their influence may not extend far enough. So it was encouraging to come across an article by a medical student who realised 'trust is a luxury that has to be earned' and questioned why some students are expected to go against guidelines and perform 'all manner of examinations on patients under general anaesthesia without their permission'.[95] I could only wonder at the conflict they must experience.

If students and healthcare professionals had time to read only one paper, they could do worse than choose 'Truth may hurt but deceit hurts more: communication in palliative care'.[18] In my opinion, the evidenced-based arguments it contains could apply equally well to all cancer patients, not just those having palliative care.

Even as I voiced patient concerns, I commiserated with staff at the increasing pressures put upon them by targets, directives, shortages and mountainous paperwork. By 2007, wholesale ward and hospital closures, staff redundancies and curtailed services were so common,[96] I felt obliged to describe myself as 'not only cancer campaigner, but NHS staff supporter'.

I had gained a deep appreciation of doctors' and nurses' difficulties and had great admiration for those who did not cling to power. And I'd learned that if some of them stood too far back, perhaps it was because they cared *too* much. They were, after all, only human, though sometimes they had to be superhuman.[51]

Chapter 59

Despite the many improvements, and perhaps inevitably, the same cancer issues continue to be raised.[97,98] Appropriate referral continues to be a contentious area, for example, a report from the National Audit Office (NAO) in 2004[99] showed only two thirds of patients who were subsequently diagnosed with cancer had been referred 'urgently' by their GP, so they may have had longer waits for assessment by a consultant. And while cancer survival rates were higher, progress varied by cancer and by locality. Improving cancer services is an ongoing, Herculean task.

In 2006, an audit of UK cancer patients showed 87% wanted to receive all possible information, whether good or bad, but were still not getting sufficient information, even when treatments could affect sexual well-being and result in near-total impotency.[100]

Although there has been growing recognition of the need for appropriate communication skills teaching and training and of the perceived benefits for both clinicians and patients,[101] poor communication with patients continues to be the most common cause of complaints against doctors.

There are plenty of recent patient stories to demonstrate that issues of pain relief, consent, communication and access have yet to be addressed: the gynaecological cancer out-patient whose colposcopist started removing post-radiotherapy internal scar-tissue without analgesia or anaesthesia – and carried on, despite her screams of, "Stop! Stop!" and protests from a specialist nurse. (For more examples of unacceptable practice in colposcopy clinics see website about cervical cancer: www.jotrust.co.uk.); the patient who was told her cancer was 'serious, but treatable' and thought this meant 'worrying, but curable'. Shortly afterwards she had a stroke and learned her prognosis as a by-line from another doctor. "We could treat you for this stroke," he said, "but before it could take effect you'd be dead from the cancer"; the 2 patients whose bowel cancers were found following routine oncology check-ups, after their GPs had treated them with pain killers for a year; the lady (a health professional) who was diagnosed with a brain tumour in 2006 but had to wait more than 4 months for an operation. Even as late as 2007, some gynaecological patients were not being told how treatment might affect their body or sexual functioning, and were not being issued with vaginal dilators.

These examples are drawn not from the wider cancer community, but from a small, local circle of friends, and are just a few of the many I could quote.

So it is heartening when NHS staff, whose own family or friends have had bad experiences of healthcare, admit to shortfalls and try to raise awareness among their colleagues.[102]

If there is no room for complacency, there is certainly room for celebrating progress to date. Medical journals increasingly invite patient contributions and even devote whole issues to the patient perspective.[103] Patients' testimonies are being heard and increasingly acted upon and when patients speak out,[104] they may also be supporting healthcare professionals by raising *their* concerns.[105,106] Raising debate may prompt meetings between interested parties and enable improvements to be set in motion.[107,108] Such loose 'partnerships' complement user involvement in service planning and implementation.

Encouragingly, the whole cancer community now seems geared up to improving services. Each edition of *Cancer Action News*, the newsletter of the Department of Health Cancer Action Team, shares new initiatives and the concept of user involvement seems to be well embedded as key to patient-centred services. The new Cancer Reform Strategy[109] promises a new era of improvements to services and care beyond treatment.

DISCUSSION

What needed to change?

Every cancer patient should be treated by a multidisciplinary team (MDT). Patients should be invited to MDT meetings.

Patient information about treatments should contain an index of side effects and complications (1 in 10: very common – 1 in 1000,000: very rare) to help patients interpret risk, as features in the Royal College of Anaesthetists' excellent series of booklets, for example 'Anaesthesia Explained'.[110] (An Australian radiotherapy consent form is very honest about potential side-effects: http://ambulance.nsw.gov.au/quality/correct/docs/radio_consent_NCCI.doc)

Every cancer patient should have access to palliative care, if necessary, throughout their disease and for late treatment effects.

Adult patients can be as vulnerable as children. Adequate pain relief should be offered, whatever the inconvenience.

Doctors need to be honest, or patients are likely to be drawn into colluding in 'false optimism'[111] and realise the truth too late.

Cancer patients should be assessed for psychological morbidity, which may appear during or after treatment.

Communication needs to improve so that patients, and every clinician involved in their care, understand their situation.

Patients need to be told in advance about early and late side effects and receive necessary support and care. The intimate side of a relationship can be as important to an older person as to a young one.

Simply asking patients if they have 'any problems' may appease clinicians' consciences, but fails patients.

'Information Prescriptions' which would give patients individually tailored information seem a good idea, but plans to tell cancer patients what symptoms to look out for once treatment has finished (patient-initiated follow-up) as a replacement for hospital follow-up consultations smacks of 'Do-it-yourself' NHS.

'Tread softly, because you tread on my dreams'
WB Yeats

Chapter 60

Eighteen years later I am still here, grateful for the treatment and expertise of the clinicians who saved my life (who knows, maybe the extra stress of fighting for information helped kick cancer into touch!) and thankful for the opportunities that resulted. What have I learned? Patient/doctor trust is essential to healing body and mind. By sharing information (power) honestly, good clinicians become 'great'.

To show compassion is the greatest gift.

Over the years, having a 'voice' and discovering health professionals with patient-centred views who seemed to be seeking to make medicine trustworthy[112] definitely helped the psychological healing process. Those who had learned it was not necessary to sacrifice their humanity in order to distance themselves from emotional involvement unwittingly sealed a crack; each a gem stored in my virtual treasure chest. I needed that balance.

In 1998, I had been privileged to become a founder member of the Royal College of Pathologists' Lay Advisory Committee.[83] The ethos of the group, comprising 6 lay and 6 professional members, was based on equity and the level of inclusiveness was phenomenal. There was mutual trust and respect; we lay people were privy to the most confidential College information and the group became integral to College working. We sat on College committees, spoke at College conferences, wrote articles and patient information, contributed to College responses to consultation documents and were invited to sumptuous annual dinners. Later, as Chair, I also attended College Council meetings.

It had been quite a culture shock to be given high levels of responsibility, to be assigned, immediately, to a national working group and have my views on sensitive issues accepted and used in national guidelines[113] and, with another lay member, co-write the accompanying patient information booklet and consent form.

I was fortunate to be asked to review a remarkable book, *Skills for Communicating with Patients,*[12] by Jonathan Silverman, Suzanne

Kurtz and Juliet Draper, for the College journal, *The Bulletin*; 'remarkable' in that the authors offer a rich, *evidence-based*, step-by-step formula for improving the communication skills training of doctors at all levels. As I turned the pages, I wanted to shout, "Yes! Yes! Yes!" Even without evidence, from my patient experiences and counselling knowledge, I could recognise the wisdom in those pages. I expressed the wish that this book (and its companion) could be used in all medical schools: surely medical education would be turned on its head, to the advantage of both patients and doctors.

The profound experience of working alongside compassionate clinicians to effect change (and similar involvement within the Royal College of General Practitioners), weighted the scales for me. The success of the partnership was due largely to the acceptance shown by our professional colleagues, and in particular to the founding Chair, Dr Helen Williams (currently Vice President). She joined the many 'good guys' in my 'treasure chest' and, with a stroke of the pen, turned the key on invading ghosts.

Her memorable words could well be adopted as a national motto for all NHS patient/professional partnership groups. They epitomise the attitude essential to the achievement of genuine user involvement and patient-centred services. They are my hope for the future:

'We need people who do not doubt our good intentions, but are prepared to tell us things others are not.'[114]

Now I feel lucky.

References

1 Audit Commission. *What Seems to be the Matter: Communication between hospitals and patients.* London: HMSO; 1993.
2 Wesley M. *Not That Sort of Girl.* London: Macmillan; 1987.
3 Walker G, Bradburn J, Maher J. *Breaking Bad News.* London: King's Fund Publishing, London; 1996.
4 Barnett MM. Effect of breaking bad news on patients' perceptions of doctors. *J R Soc Med.* 2002; **95**: 343–7.
5 Tattersall MHN, Butow PN, Griffin A, *et al.* The take-home message: patients prefer consultation tapes to summary letters. *J Clin Oncol.* 1994; **12**: 1305–11.
6 Ong LML, Visser MRM, Lammes FB, *et al.* Effect of providing cancer patients with the audiotaped initial consultation on satisfaction, recall, and quality of life: a randomized double-blind study. *J Clin Oncol.* 2000; **18**: 3052–60.

7   *The Red Shoes*. Film, written, produced and directed by Michael Powell and Emeric Pressburger. Distributed by Eagle-Lion Distributors (UK), Eagle-Lion Films Inc. (US). Release date September 1948.

8   Kesey K. *One Flew Over the Cuckoo's Nest*. London: Macmillan; 1973.

9   Papillon J, Montbarbon JF. Epidemoid carcinoma of the anal canal: a series of 276 cases. *Dis Colon Rectum*. 1987; **30**: 324–33. In: Bosset JF, Pavy JJ, Roelofsen F, Bartelink H. Combined radiotherapy and chemotherapy for anal cancer. Correspondence. *Lancet*. 1997; **349**: 205.

10 O'Connor AM, Rostom A, Fiset V, *et al*. Decision aids for patients facing health treatment or screening decisions: systematic review. *BMJ*. 1999; **319**: 731–4.

11 Say RE, Thomson R. The importance of patient preferences in treatment decisions – challenges for doctors. *BMJ*. 2003; **327**: 542–5.

12 Silverman J, Kurtz S, Draper J. *Skills for Communicating with Patients*. Oxford: Radcliffe Medical Press; 1998.

13 General Medical Council. *Seeking Patients' Consent: the ethical considerations*. London: GMC; 1998. Available at: www.gmc-uk.org/guidance/ethical_guidance/index.asp (accessed 20 September 2007).

14 Garry A. Palliative care. In: Baker MR (ed.) *Modernising Cancer Services*. Oxford: Radcliffe Medical Press; 2002, pp.175–91.

15 Dickinson D, Theo Raynor DK, Kennedy JG, *et al*. What information do patients need about medicines? *BMJ*. 2003; **327**: 861–4.

16 The Royal College of Radiologists' Clinical Oncology Patients' Liaison Group. *Making Your Radiotherapy Service More Patient-Friendly*. London: The Royal College of Radiologists; 1999. Available at: www.rcr.ac.uk/index.asp?PageID=149&PublicationID=256 (accessed 24 November 2007).

17 The Royal Marsden NHS Foundation Trust. *Radiotherapy patient information booklet*. London: The Royal Marsden NHS Foundation Trust. Available at: www.royalmarsden.nhs.uk/RMH/cancer/treatment of cancer/treatmenttypes/radiotherapy/radiotherapytreatment.htm (accessed 16 November 2007).

18 Fallowfield LJ, Jenkins VA, Beveridge HA. Truth may hurt but deceit hurts more: communication in palliative care. *Pall Med*. 2002; **16**: 297–303.

19 The Royal Marsden NHS Foundation Trust. *Living with Cancer: eating well*. London: The Royal Marsden NHS Foundation Trust. Available at: www.royalmarsden.nhs.uk/RMH/cancer/livingwithcancer/eatingwell.htm (accessed 16 September 2007).

20 Carmichael R. Help! I'm dying. *Oncol Newsletter. J York Reg Cancer Org*. 1993; **12**: 13–14.

21 Jelley D, Walker C. Sharing information with patients. In: Harrison J, Innes R, van Zwanenberg T (eds) *Rebuilding Trust in Healthcare*. Oxford: Radcliffe Medical Press; 2003, pp.131–42.

22 The Royal College of Radiologists' Clinical Radiology Patients' Liaison Group. *Making Your Radiology Service More Patient-Friendly*. Board of the Faculty of Clinical Radiology. London: The Royal College of

Radiologists; 2000. Updated 2007. Available at: www.rcr.ac.uk/docs/radiology/pdf/radiofriendly.pdf (accessed 24 November 2007).

23 Skinner B, Springham S. Web Alert: finding high-quality patient information resources online. *Qual Prim Care.* 2007; **15**: 247–51.

24 www.labtestsonline.org.uk (accessed 9 March 2008).

25 Cancerbackup. *Freedom from Pain Charter.* London: Cancerbackup; 2001. (Launched at the Royal Society of Medicine, 9 April 2001.)

26 *Freedom from Pain Conference: current issues in cancer pain management.* Cancerbackup in association with Mark Allen International Communications Ltd. Institute of Physics, Portland Place, London, 12 June 2001.

27 Coulter A. Paternalism or partnership? Patients have grown up and there's no going back. *BMJ.* 1999; **319**: 719–20.

28 Stern V. Gynaecological examination post-Ledward: a private matter. *Lancet.* 2001; **358**: 1896–8.

29 General Medical Council. *Duties of a Doctor Registered with the General Medical Council: good medical practice.* London: GMC; 2006. Available at: www.gmc-uk.org/guidance/good_medical_practice/duties_of_a_doctor.asp (accessed 22 September 2007).

30 General Medical Council. *Intimate Examinations.* London: GMC; 2001. Available at: www.gmc-uk.org/guidance/current/library/intimate_examinations.asp (accessed 22 September 2007).

31 Helman C. Introduction: The Healing Bond. In: Helman C (ed.) *Doctors and Patients: an anthology.* Oxford: Radcliffe Medical Press; 2003, p.9.

32 Carroll L. *Alice's Adventures in Wonderland.* Chapter 2: Pool of Tears, p.20; Chapter 8: The Queen's Croquet Ground, pp.94–107; Chapter 1: Down the Rabbit Hole, p.17. London and Glasgow: Collins Clear-type Press.

33 Blennerhassett M. The pain of the gentle touch. *Health Serv J.* 1996; **5497**: 25.

34 Blennerhassett M. Deadly charades. *BMJ.* 1998; **316**: 1890–1.

35 Macmillan Cancer Relief. *The Unclaimed Millions.* London: Macmillan Cancer Relief; 2004.

36 Mackenzie JW. Daycase anaesthesia and anxiety. *Anaes.* 1989; **44**: 437–40.

37 Lack JA, Rollin A-M, Thoms G, et al. *Raising the Standard: information for patients.* London: The Royal College of Anaesthetists; 2003.

38 Rose D. Foreign doctors face competence inquiry. *The Times.* 10 August 2007, p.1.

39 Tanner G, Myers P. Secondary-primary care communication: impressions of the quality of consultant communication with specific regard to cancer patients. *Prim Hlth Care Res Develop.* 2002; **3**: 23–8.

40 Kipling R. The Cat that Walked by Himself. In: *The Complete Just So Stories.* London: Little, Brown and Company; 1993, pp.125–37.

41 Shepard EH. Winnie the Pooh. In: *In Which a House is Built at Pooh Corner for Eeyore.* London: Methuen; 1926, Chapter 1.

42 CancerWise. *Patient faces recurrence fear with action* (March 2005). Available at: www.cancerwise.org/March_2005/display.cfm?id=A71C9B (accessed 20 September 2007).

43 Kubler Ross E. *On Death and Dying. What the dying have to teach*

doctors, nurses, clergy and their own families. London: Routledge; 1989.

44 Fallowfield LJ, Rodway A, Baum M. What are the psychological factors influencing attendance, non-attendance and re-attendance at a breast screening centre? *J R Soc Med*. 1990; 83(9): 547–51.

45 Mitchel V. With your clothes on. *LinkUp*. 1991; 24. London: CancerLink.

46 Measham Medical Unit, High Street, Measham, Near Swadlincote, Derbyshire DE12 7HR. Tel: 01530 270667. Email: mmu@tesco.net

47 Jencks M. Joy of life in the darkest shadow. *Daily Telegraph*. 20 July 1995, p.2.

48 The All Party Parliamentary Group on Breast Cancer. Support and Help Group Awards Certificate. July 1999.

49 Penny Brohn Cancer Care, Chapel Pill Lane, Pill, Bristol BS20 0HH. Tel: 01275 370 100. National Telephone Helpline: 0845 123 23 10. Fax: 01275 370 101. Email: info@pennybrohn.org. Website: www. pennybrohncancercare.org (accessed 8 September 2007).

50 Etchells R. The patient's perspective. In: Harrison J, Innes R, van Zwanenberg T (eds) *Rebuilding Trust in Healthcare*. Oxford: Radcliffe Medical Press; 2003, pp.5–14.

51 Gibson H. Personal view. The system must change. *Student BMJ*. 1997; 5: 219.

52 Russell J. *Keeping Abreast*. York: Insight Press; 1998.

53 Blennerhassett M. So why don't cancer patients complain? *LinkUp*. 1995; 39: 12–13. London: CancerLink.

54 Blennerhassett M. Training doctors: what are your rights as a patient? *LinkUp*. 1996; 44: 20–1. London: CancerLink.

55 Taylor RE, United Kingdom Co-ordinating Committee for Cancer Research Anal Cancer Trial Update. *Oncology Newsletter*. 1991; Summer: 6.

56 UKCCCR Anal Cancer Trial Working Party. Epidermoid anal cancer: results from the UKCCCR Anal Cancer Trial Working Party. *Lancet*. 1996; 348: 1049–54.

57 UKCCCR Anal Cancer Trial. *UKCCCR Anal Cancer Trial Winter Newsletter*. London: UKCCCR Anal Cancer Working Party; 1996.

58 UKCCCR Anal Cancer Trial. *Protocol Modifications. Recommendations on Prevention and Monitoring Toxic Reactions*. London: UKCCCR Anal Cancer Working Party; 1989.

59 UKCCCR Anal Cancer Trial. Results of the UKCCCR Phase III Anal Cancer Trial: The Parallel Quality of Life Study. *UKCCCR Anal Cancer Trial Winter Newsletter*. London: UKCCCR Anal Cancer Working Party; 1996.

60 Tattersall M, Ellis P. Communication is a vital part of care. *BMJ*. 1998; 316: 1891–2.

61 Metcalfe D. Doctors and patients should be fellow travellers. *BMJ*. 1998; 316: 1892–3.

62 Steel N. Specialist training should include communication skills. *BMJ*. 1999; 318: 60.

63 Taylor RE. Hostility can be a barrier to effective communication. *BMJ.* 1999; **318**: 60.

64 *Pulse* (York District Hospital in-house magazine); April 2000, p.10.

65 Williamson C. Withholding policies from patients restricts their autonomy. *BMJ.* 2005; **331**: 1078–80.

66 Lacroix A, Jacquemet S, Assal JP, Benroubi M. The patients' voice; testimonies from patients suffering from chronic disease. *Patient Educ Coun.* 1995; **26**(1–3): 293–9.

67 Stead ML, Brown JM, Fallowfield L, Selby P. Lack of communication between healthcare professionals and women with ovarian cancer about sexual issues. *Br J Cancer.* 2003; **88**: 666–71.

68 Moffatt CJ, Franks PJ, Doherty DC, *et al.* Lymphoedema: an underestimated problem. *Q J Med.* 2003; **96**: 731–8.

69 *The Lymphoedema Framework Journal.* 2003; Edition 1: Autumn.

70 National Forum of Gynaecological Oncology Nurses. *Best Practice Guidelines on the Use of Vaginal Dilators in Women Receiving Pelvic Radiotherapy.* Amersham, Bucks: National Forum of Gynaecological Oncology Nurses; Woodstock, Oxon: Owen Mumford; 2005.

71 National Institute for Clinical Excellence. *Guidance on Cancer Services: improving supportive and palliative care for adults with cancer.* London: NICE; 2004.

72 Blennerhassett M. What cancer patients need. In: Baker MR (ed.) *Modernising Cancer Services.* Oxford: Radcliffe Medical Press; 2002, p.158.

73 General Medical Council. *Tomorrow's Doctors. Recommendations on Undergraduate Medical Education.* London: GMC; 1993.

74 Child JA. Editorial: Patient power. *Oncol Newsletter. J York Reg Cancer Org.* 1995; **20**: 2.

75 Lane R. Communication. *Oncol Newsletter. J York Reg Cancer Org.* 1994; **Spring**: 6–7.

76 Jenkins V, Fallowfield L. Can communication skills training alter physicians' beliefs and behaviour in clinics? *J Clin Oncol;* **20**: 765–9.

77 NHS Executive. *A Policy Framework for Commissioning Cancer Services: A Report of the Expert Advisory Group on Cancer to the Chief Medical Officer of England and Wales* (Calman-Hine Report). London: DoH; 1995.

78 Lakhani M, Dale J. Patient involvement in clinical governance. *J Clin Gov.* 1999; **17**: 99–101.

79 Coulter A. Editorial: Paternalism or partnership? Patients have grown up – and there's no going back. *BMJ.* 1999; **319**: 719–20.

80 Hine D. *Principles and Paradoxes in Modern Healthcare.* London: The Nuffield Trust; 2007.

81 Tallis R. Hippocratic Oaths. Medicine and its discontents. In: Hine D. *Principles and Paradoxes in Modern Healthcare.* London: The Nuffield Trust; 2007.

82 NHS Executive. *NHS Plan 2000.* London: DoH; 2000.

83 NHS Executive. *NHS Cancer Plan 2000.* London: DoH; 2000.

84 Williams H. Patients and pathologists. *ACP News.* 2000; **Summer**: 30–2.

85 National Council for Hospice and Palliative Care Services. Specialist

Palliative care: a statement of definitions. Occasional paper 8. London: NCHSPCS; 1995. Quoted in: Garry A. Palliative care. In: Baker MR (ed.) *Modernising Cancer Services*. Oxford: Radcliffe Medical Press; 2002, pp.175–89.

86 Dickinson D, Theo Raynor DK. Ask the patients – they may want to know more than you think. *BMJ*. 2003; **327**: 861.

87 General Medical Council. *Maintaining Boundaries*. London: GMC; 2006. Available at: www.gmcuk.org/guidance/current/library/maintaining_boundaries.asp (accessed 16 November 2007).

88 Macmillan Cancer Relief, NHS Modernisation Agency, National Cancer Action Team. *Cancer in Primary Care: a guide to good practice*. London: DoH; 2004.

89 Hanley B, Stanley K. *Yesterday's Women. The story of RAGE*. TwoCan Associates research on behalf of Macmillan Cancer Support. London: Macmillan Cancer Support; 2006.

90 NHS Direct. *Health Encyclopaedia: Radiotherapy*. Available at: www.nhsdirect.nhs.uk/articles/article.aspx?articleId=309&sec (accessed 16 November 2007).

91 Measham Medical Unit, High Street, Measham, Near Swadlincote, Derbyshire DE12 7HR. Tel: 01530 270667. Email: mmu@tesco.net

92 Randev P. Editorial: Drug data records – a new hazard. *Prescriber*. 2004; **15**: 8.

93 Baker M. Correspondence: Drug data records. *Prescriber*. 2004; **15**(14).

94 Fallowfield LJ. *Truth Hurts But Deceit Hurts More: Talking About Cancer*. The Sixth Annual Lecture, Cancer Education and Communication Group, Yorkshire Cancer Organisation, 4 December 1995.

95 Shaw ASJ. Do we really know the law about students and patient consent? *BMJ*. 2005; **331**: 522.

96 Mandelstam M. *Betraying the NHS. Health Abandoned*. London: Jessica Kingsley Publishers; 2006.

97 The Picker Institute Europe. *At a crossroads without signposts*. Available at: www.pickereurope.org/Filestore/Publications/Information_access_final_web.pdf (accessed 17 September 2007).

98 NHS Centre for Reviews and Dissemination. Informing, communicating and sharing decisions with people who have cancer. *Effect Hlth Care Bull*. 2000; **6**(6).

99 National Audit Office. *Tackling Cancer in England: saving more lives*. Report by the Comptroller and Auditor General. London: NAO; 2004.

100 Cox A, Jenkins V, Catt S, *et al*. Information needs and experiences: an audit of UK cancer patients. *Euro J Oncol Nurs*. 2006; **10**: 263–72.

101 Fallowfield L, Jenkins V. Communicating sad, bad, and difficult news in medicine. *Lancet*. 2004; **363**: 312–19.

102 Llewellyn L. On listening to patients. *Hlth Serv J*. 2006; **5 January**: 15.

103 Blennerhassett M. Challenges for primary care in the age of the autonomous patient. *Qual Prim Care*. 2007; **15**(4): 201-6.

104 Tylko K, Blennerhassett M. How the NHS could better protect the safety of radiotherapy patients. *Health Care Risk Report*. 2006; **12**: 18–19.

105 Williams MV. Radiotherapy near misses, incidents and errors: radiotherapy incident at Glasgow. *Clin Oncol.* 2007; **19**: 1–3.

106 Donaldson L. Reducing harm from radiotherapy. *BMJ.* 2007; **334**: 272.

107 Donaldson L. *Chief Medical Officer's Annual Report 2006.* Available from: www.dh.gov.uk/en/Publicationsandstatistics/Publications/AnnualReports/DH076817 (accessed 16 September 2007).

108 Williams M. Radiotherapy: Developing a world class service (National Radiotherapy Advisory Group update). *Cancer Action.* Newsletter from the Cancer Action Team. London: DoH; 2007, p.8.

109 Department of Health. *The Cancer Reform Strategy.* London: DoH; 2007. Available from: www.dh.gov.uk/ (accessed 4 December 2007). Hard copies available from: DoH Publications Orderline, PO Box 777, London SE1 6XH. Tel: 0870 555 5455.

110 Royal College of Anaesthetists. *Anaesthesia Explained.* London: Royal College of Anaesthetists and Association of Anaesthetists of Great Britain and Ireland; 2002.

111 The A, Hak T, Koeter G, *et al.* Collusion in doctor–patient communication about imminent death: an ethnographic study. *BMJ.* 2000; **321**: 1376–81.

112 Irvine D. *The Doctor's Tale: Professionalism and public trust.* Oxford: Radcliffe Medical Press; 2003.

113 Royal College of Pathologists. *Guidelines for the Retention of Tissues and Organs at Post Mortem Examination.* London: RCP; 2000.

114 Williams H. Registrar's Report. *Bull Roy Coll Pathol.* 2003; **124**: 33–4.

Further reading

Advisory Committee on Breast Cancer Screening, Austoker J, Beral V, Berrington A, Blanks RG. Screening for breast cancer in England: past and future. *J Med Screen.* 2006; **13**: 59–61.

Baker MR (ed.) *Modernising Cancer Services.* Oxford: Radcliffe Medical Press; 2002.

Barrows HS, Pickell GC. *Developing Clinical Problem-Solving Skills. A Guide to More Effective Diagnosis and Treatment.* New York: WW Norton and Company Inc.; 1991.

Batt S. *Patient No More.* Charlottetown, PEI, Canada: Gynergy Books; 1994.

Bolton G (ed.) *Dying, Bereavement and the Healing Arts.* London: Jessica Kingsley Publishers; 2008.

Brennan J, Sheard T. Psychosocial support and therapy in cancer care. *Euro J Pall Care.* 1(3): 136–9.

Evans I, Thornton H, Chalmers I. *Testing Treatments. Better Research for Better Healthcare.* London: The British Library; 2006. Now freely available from: testingtreatments@jameslindlibrary.org

Gawande A. *Better: A surgeon's notes on performance.* London: Picador; 2007.

General Medical Council. *Tomorrow's Doctors. Recommendations on Undergraduate Medical Education.* London: GMC; 1993.

Hanley B, Stanley K. *Yesterday's Women. The story of RAGE.* TwoCan Associates research on behalf of Macmillan Cancer Support. London: Macmillan Cancer Support; 2006.

Harrison J, Innes R, van Zwanenberg T (eds) *Rebuilding Trust in Healthcare.* Oxford: Radcliffe Medical Press; 2003.

Helman C (ed.) *Doctors and Patients: an anthology.* Oxford: Radcliffe Medical Press; 2003.

Hine D. *Principles and Paradoxes in Modern Healthcare.* London: The Nuffield Trust; 2007.

Irvine D. *The Doctor's Tale: Professionalism and public trust.* Oxford: Radcliffe Medical Press; 2003.

Lack JA, Rollin A-M, Thoms G, *et al. Raising the Standard: Information for patients.* London: The Royal College of Anaesthetists; 2003.

Lee E. *A Good Death: A guide for patients and carers facing terminal illness at home.* London: Rosendale Press; 1995.

Mandelstam M. *Betraying the NHS. Health Abandoned.* London: Jessica Kingsley Publishers; 2006.

NHS Executive. Principles for information giving. A view from a workshop of patients' organisations sponsored by the Quality & Consumer Unit of the NHS Executive Headquarters. *Patient's Charter News,* Issue 20, June 1995.

Plant J. *Your Life in Your Hands. Understanding, Preventing and Overcoming Breast Cancer.* London: Virgin Books; 2001.

Poulson J. Bitter pills to swallow. *N Engl J Med.* 1998; **338**: 1844–6.

Rendell A. Understanding dying: the patient as manager. *Information Exchange.* 2001; **32**: 2–13.

Rendell A. Management theory and the patient's potential. *Information Exchange.* 2001; **33**: 14–15.

Rendell A. Can't get no satisfaction? *Information Exchange.* 2001; **34**: 12–13.

Russell J. *Keeping Abreast.* York: Insight Press; 1998.

Sandkühler J. Fear the pain. *Lancet.* 2002; **360**: 426.

Silverman J, Kurtz S, Draper J. *Skills for Communicating with Patients.* Oxford: Radcliffe Medical Press; 1998.

Skevington SM. *Psychology of Pain.* Chichester: John Wiley and Sons; 1995.

The National Cancer Alliance. *'Patient-Centred Cancer Services'? What Patients Say.* Oxford: NCA; 1996.

Worden JW. *Grief Counselling and Grief Therapy.* London: Tavistock/Routledge Publications; 1982.

Printed and bound by CPI Group (UK) Ltd, Croydon, CR0 4YY

22/10/2024

01777622-0001